ALLEN CARR'S
EASY WAY
FOR WOMEN TO
LOSE
WEIGHT

SIRIUS

To our amazing team of Senior Allen Carr's Easyway Therapists around the world

Thanks also to Tim Glynne-Jones for additional editorial input

SIRIUS

This edition published in 2022 by Sirius Publishing, a division of
Arcturus Publishing Limited,
26/27 Bickels Yard, 151–153 Bermondsey Street,
London SE1 3HA

ISBN: 978-1-78428-263-9
AD004834US

Printed in the UK

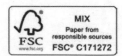

MIX
Paper from
responsible sources
FSC® C171272

ALLEN CARR

Allen Carr was a chain-smoker for over 30 years. In 1983, after countless failed attempts to quit, he went from 100 cigarettes a day to zero without suffering withdrawal pangs, without using willpower, and without putting on weight. He realized that he had discovered what the world had been waiting for—the easy way to stop smoking—and embarked on a mission to help cure the world's smokers.

As a result of the phenomenal success of his method, he gained an international reputation as the world's leading expert on stopping smoking and his network of centers now spans the globe. His first book, *Allen Carr's Easy Way to Stop Smoking*, has sold more than 14 million copies, remains a global best-seller, and has been published in over 40 different languages. Hundreds of thousands of smokers have successfully quit at Allen Carr's Easyway Centers where they guarantee you'll find it easy to stop or you'll get your money back.

Allen Carr's Easyway method has been successfully applied to a host of issues including weight control, alcohol, debt, and other addictions. A list of Allen Carr centers appears at the back of this book. If you require any assistance or if you have any questions, please do not hesitate to contact your nearest center.

For more information about Allen Carr's Easyway, please visit **www.allencarr.com**

Allen Carr's Easyway

The key that will set you free

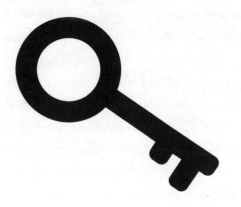

CONTENTS

PREFACE

I had struggled with my weight since childhood. I remember being told by my older brothers that I was fat when I was five years old. I was told by a school nurse to stop eating yogurts when I was eight because I was overweight! Strangely enough, when I look at pictures of myself from those times, I was positively skinny by today's standards.

Still, those words stuck with me and for the next 35 years my weight went up and down. It's no exaggeration to say that I was completely obsessed by food and my looks. No event was untouched by my mental struggle with eating. Every day a huge chunk of my thinking was taken up with how fat I was, when and what I could eat next, which clothes to wear to conceal my weight and, above all, what other people thought of me—how weak, trapped, and stupid I felt. Food made me miserable and yet I couldn't see a way out.

I visited Allen Carr's Easyway center in Raynes Park, London on two occasions in 1997. Firstly to get free from smoking and a few months later to escape the alcohol trap. On each occasion, I emerged six hours later completely free and and I haven't felt the desire for a cigarette or a drink since. When Allen applied his method to weight loss, I was excited to try it. Like with smoking and drinking, he made me realize that I had been completely hooked on an idea that certain types of food were playing a role in my life that they simply weren't. Since I accepted the reality that the fattening foods that we all tend to think of as our favorites aren't really the amazing pleasure or crutch that we're led to believe, and that the foods that are best for us also taste the best, my life has improved in every way.

Mealtimes are so much more enjoyable because I'm eating foods that are nutritious and taste great. They satisfy me without making me feel bloated. I don't feel envious of what other people are eating—I can see they're in the same trap I was in. When I get an invitation to a special event, it's no longer overshadowed by the dread of finding something to wear. These days I actually look forward to shopping for clothes. All that time, headspace, and energy that were previously consumed by my eating issues are now spent ENJOYING LIFE.

I will always be grateful to Allen for the help he gave me and I was delighted to be given the opportunity to work for Easyway and help other people to benefit as I had. Allen originally devised his method to help people quit smoking and it was—and still is—a phenomenal success.

More than 400,000 people have attended Easyway centers in over 50 countries and Allen Carr's Easyway books have been translated into more than 40 languages, have sold more than 16 million copies, and the method is estimated to have cured 30 million people. This success has been achieved not through slick advertising or smart marketing campaigns but through the personal recommendations of the millions of people who have succeeded with the method. Allen Carr's Easyway has spread all over the world for one reason alone: BECAUSE IT WORKS.

The Easy Way for Women to Lose Weight addresses a problem that is by no means unique to women but is, nevertheless, one that traps women in a particularly aggressive way, such is the focus on body image these days. The beauty of this method is that it makes eating a pleasure first and foremost, with the happy consequence of keeping you looking and feeling great without having to make sacrifices or put yourself through punishing exercise routines.

Thanks to Allen Carr, I feel happy and healthy in a way I simply could not have imagined before I discovered Easyway. I am sure that this method will change your life just as it has changed mine.

Colleen Dwyer
Senior Therapist, Allen Carr's Easyway

INTRODUCTION

By John Dicey, Global CEO & Senior Therapist, Allen Carr's Easyway

For a third of a century Allen Carr chain-smoked 60 to 100 cigarettes a day. With the exception of acupuncture, he'd tried all the conventional methods to quit, using willpower, nicotine replacement, hypnotherapy, substitutes, and other gimmicks, all without success.

As he describes it: "It was like being between the devil and the deep blue sea. I desperately wanted to quit, but whenever I tried I was utterly miserable. No matter how long I survived without a cigarette, I never felt completely free. It was as if I had lost my best friend, my crutch, my character, my very personality. In those days I believed there were such types as addictive personalities or confirmed smokers, and because my family were all heavy smokers, I believed that there was something in our genes that meant we couldn't enjoy life or cope with stress without smoking."

Eventually he gave up even trying to quit, believing: once a smoker, always a smoker. Then he discovered something which motivated him to try again:

"I went overnight from 100 cigarettes a day to zero—without any bad temper or sense of loss, void, or depression. On the contrary, I actually enjoyed the process. I knew I was already a nonsmoker even before I had extinguished my final cigarette and I've never had the slightest urge to smoke since."

It didn't take Allen long to realize that he had discovered a method of quitting that would enable any smoker to quit

- EASILY, IMMEDIATELY, AND PERMANENTLY
- WITHOUT USING WILLPOWER, AIDS, SUBSTITUTES OR GIMMICKS
- WITHOUT SUFFERING DEPRESSION OR WITHDRAWAL SYMPTOMS
- WITHOUT GAINING WEIGHT

After using his smoking friends and relatives as guinea pigs to test the method, he gave up his lucrative profession as a qualified accountant and set up a center to help other smokers to quit.

He called his method "EASYWAY," and so successful has it been that there are now Allen Carr's Easyway centers in more than 150 cities in 50 countries worldwide. Best-selling books based on his method are now translated into over 40 languages, with more being added each year.

It quickly became clear to Allen that his method could be applied to other problems of addiction. The method has helped tens of millions of people quit smoking, alcohol, and other drugs, as well as to stop gambling, stop overeating, and stop overspending.

The method works by unraveling the misconceptions that make people believe that they get some benefit from the very thing that's harming them.

This book applies the method to the issue of losing weight and unlike other methods it does not require willpower.

Too good to be true? All you have to do is read the book in its entirety, follow all the instructions, and you cannot fail.

I'm aware that the claims of the method's success might appear far-fetched or exaggerated, at times even outrageous. That was certainly my reaction when I first heard them. I was incredibly fortunate to attend Allen Carr's center in London in the late 1990s—yet I did so under duress. I had agreed to go, at the request of my wife, on the understanding that when I walked out of the center and remained a smoker she would leave it at least 12 months before hassling me about stopping smoking again. No one was more surprised than me, or perhaps my wife, that Allen Carr's Easyway method set me free from my 80-a-day addiction.

I was so inspired that I hassled and harangued Allen Carr and Robin Hayley (now chairman of Allen Carr's Easyway) to let me get involved in their quest to cure the world of smoking. I was incredibly fortunate in persuading them to allow me to do so. Being trained by Allen Carr and Robin Hayley was one of the most rewarding experiences of my life. To be able to count Allen as not only my coach and mentor but also my friend was an amazing honor and privilege. Allen Carr and Robin Hayley trained me well: I personally went on to treat more than 30,000 smokers at Allen's original London center, and became part of the team that has taken Allen's method from Berlin to Bogota, from New Zealand to New York, from Sydney to Santiago.

Tasked by Allen with insuring that his legacy achieves its

full potential, we've taken Allen Carr's Easyway from videos to DVDs, from centers to apps, from computer games to audio books, to online programs and beyond. We've a long way to go, with so many addictions and issues to apply the method to, and this book plays a special part in our quest.

The honor of adding a light editorial touch to update and develop Allen's method in this book has fallen to me and the amazing Colleen Dwyer, one of the most senior Allen Carr's Easyway therapists in the world.

Editing Allen's work as we have enables us to apply the most up-to-date, cutting-edge version of his method to a whole host of issues, while inserting, where necessary, up-to-date examples and references within the text.

Follow Allen Carr's instructions and you'll find it not only easy to be the weight you want to be, but you'll actually enjoy the whole process. You won't just be free; you'll be happy to be free. That might sound too good to be true at the moment, but read on: you have nothing to lose and absolutely everything to gain. Let me pass you into the safest of hands— over to Allen Carr.

Chapter 1

DIETS DON'T WORK

The misery and frustration of trying and failing to lose weight is a particular concern for women and one that they are under constant pressure to conquer. This book will show you how to succeed easily, painlessly, and permanently.

Once upon a time, losing weight was perceived as something a woman did in order to fit into her summer dress or look good for the beach. Obesity was a condition suffered only by the unfortunate few and you could count the number of diets available on the fingers of one hand. But since the tail end of the last century the problem of being overweight has mushroomed into a global epidemic that has taken the matter of what and how we eat way above the fashion agenda and into the realms of "serious health threat."

AND IT'S WORSE FOR WOMEN!

According to the World Health Organization, the prevalence of obesity among women nearly doubled between 1980 and 2008, from 8 percent to 14 percent—one-and-a-half times the incidence among men, and it continues to rise. Unlike most global health problems, the problem is most extreme in the so-called "developed world," with a proven link between weight and wealth showing that people in the better-off regions are more prone to being overweight. In the Americas, nearly two-thirds of adults over the age of 20 are overweight and where America leads, Europe soon follows. More than half the women in Europe and the Americas combined have a weight problem.

It's something of a paradox: In a world that's become increasingly obsessed with diets and body image, particularly for women, people—and women in particular—are becoming increasingly overweight.

WHY?

FACT
According to the World Health Organization, 2.8 million people die each year as a result of being overweight or obese.

THE GENDER GAP

The obvious answer is that we eat too much and exercise too little. We drive instead of walking or biking and we spend evenings sitting in front of the TV instead of working, playing a sport or going out dancing or clubbing. In these respects we have changed over the past 100 years, but it doesn't explain why modern women are more prone to weight problems than men. Surely, it wasn't needlework and the occasional tea dance that kept women in trim a century ago!

There are physiological reasons why women are more prone to weight gain than men. On average a healthy woman carries one-and-a-half to two times as much body fat as a healthy man and requires fewer calories for each pound of body weight. Therefore, women put on weight more easily than men. Moreover, the change in women's roles within society has seen the amount of food and drink that women consume move closer to that of their male counterparts, notably the consumption of alcohol.

Back in 1980 it was unusual for women to go out drinking in the way that men did, and certainly not to consume the same sort of quantities. But the desire among women to have the same opportunities as men spilled over into cultural behaviors that have seen the amount of alcohol consumed by women increase exponentially. Regular consumption of significant amounts of alcohol is a major cause of being overweight.

Sex equality has also brought pressure. More women than ever are going out to work and having to deal with stressful careers. The increase in opportunity to build a career has not been counterbalanced by an equivalent decrease in domestic or maternal obligations, and the competition for jobs, schools, houses, etc. grows increasingly intense. Women are becoming more "time poor" with each passing year and, therefore, are relying increasingly on so-called "convenience" foods for sustenance and "comfort" foods and alcohol in an attempt to relieve the stress. In fact, these foods and drink don't relieve stress at all, they add to it, as I will explain later in the book.

More and more women are discovering the misery of being overweight and feeling powerless to do anything about it. It's an all-too-familiar story: The only way they know to alleviate the misery is to eat "comfort foods" like cookies, cakes or candy—and while they're well aware that this stuff isn't doing them any good, they just can't seem to stop.

So they turn to the other side of the problem: exercise. They join a gym or take up jogging and try to burn off those extra pounds. But what happens when they exert themselves? They get hungry and thirsty. So each exercise session makes them eat and drink more. Whichever way they turn, they seem to be caught in a trap. And you're probably not any different...

Countless diets have failed you, just as they've failed millions of overweight women, and so have the exercise regimes. You feel like a failure, too weak willed to stick to a diet or exercise regime long enough to make it work. Well I've got news for you:

DIETS DON'T WORK!

And neither does exercise, for the reason I've just explained. For exercise you need fuel. Keep fueling up with the same old junk and you will not lose weight.

It all seems so complicated, doesn't it? You're probably thinking, "If only there was an easy way to solve my weight problem, then it wouldn't matter that I don't have the willpower." Here's the next piece of good news: There is an easy way. Added to which,

YOU DON'T NEED WILLPOWER

Your inability to control your weight through dieting or exercise is nothing to do with a weakness in you. The reason you've been unable to control your weight until now is quite simply because you've been following the wrong method. Before we get on to the right method, let's examine why you want to lose weight.

> **FACT**
> Being overweight is a proven life shortener: WHO figures estimate that annually it accounts for 35.8 million lost years of healthy life among the world's population.

THE REAL DAMAGE

There are many good reasons for tackling a weight problem, not least of which is the impact it can have on your health. Proven links with raised blood pressure, cholesterol, and Type 2 diabetes have been established for years. These conditions in turn increase your risk of heart disease and stroke. As weight increases, so does the risk of contracting numerous forms of cancer, including breast cancer and cancer of the womb. If you want to lose years off your life, being overweight is a good way to go about it.

These health risks are well publicized and people are becoming more and more aware of them, yet the problem is increasing. Clearly fear of the potential health impact alone is not enough to make us change the way we eat. Just as the health warnings on cigarette packs make not the slightest difference to the smoker, when you're overweight you become adept at turning a deaf ear to the health warnings about overeating. In fact, being made to fear the consequences of overeating will actually make you more inclined to overeat.

If the one thing that appears to give you comfort in life is food, what's the one thing you'll turn to in distress? It may sound absurd, but that is the nature of the problem. It's a trap that hooks you in and makes you see things back to front.

We're all well aware of the health impact of being overweight, just as the smoker is in no doubt that continuing to smoke is causing incredible damage to their health and likely to lead to a slow, painful, premature death, but this knowledge is not enough to prevent millions of women from continuing to eat and drink junk that makes them overweight and unhappy. That's because the serious health risk is not the reason why most women want to lose weight. It's the everyday damage that being overweight does to you both physically and mentally: the feeling you get when you look in the mirror, the clothes that don't fit any more, the self-consciousness in public, the lack of energy, the shortness of breath after minimal exertion, the sense of helplessness and self-loathing every time you binge on food or drink.

In short, the health fears aren't what make you want to resolve the issue—it's simply the way being overweight makes you feel every day.

You might have your life under control in every other way, yet when it comes to what you eat and drink you've developed a sneaking suspicion that you're not the one in control. Every time you try to curb it, you find yourself going back for more. Have you ever been in that situation when you allow yourself a piece of chocolate or a cookie and before you know it you've eaten the whole package? You don't even remember what most of those chocolates or cookies tasted like.

This is a classic sign that you're in a trap.

LOOKING FOR A WAY OUT

So why is it so hard to resist a package of cookies? No one's holding a gun to your head and forcing you to eat them. When you stop to think about it, they're not even that tasty. You know they're not good for you. And you know that if you eat them, you'll feel miserable afterward.

YET YOU STILL EAT THE WHOLE PACKAGE!

With all this common sense in your head it should be pretty easy to resist eating even one cookie, let alone the whole package. Why does it seem to require such a gargantuan effort? And why, however you try, do you never seem to be able to sustain it?

We've used the package of cookies as a common example. You might not have a weakness for cookies, it might be something else, something you just can't resist: most likely quite a few things fall into that category.

Whatever it is, you'll be familiar with the problem. You know you don't need it. You know it's not good for you, yet a voice in your head keeps telling you that you want it.

Why can't you just take over control and silence that voice in your head?

Earlier I described being overweight as a trap. Imagine you're in a prison with walls ten feet thick, one tiny slit of light high up out of reach, and the only way out is a heavy iron door that you've been told is almost impossible to open.

The first thing you do is try to open that door but, finding it too heavy for you to budge, you soon give up and mope about, convinced that escape is indeed impossible. That's the state that people find themselves in after failed attempts to diet: trapped in a prison from which they're convinced they cannot escape —convinced because they've tried and failed. What they don't realize is that they've been following the wrong method.

This method is going to show you that there is a way out of that prison and, what's more, it's easy. Ask yourself why you think it has to be hard. It's because other people have told you so and because you've tried and failed yourself! But you only failed because you were using the wrong method. And so have all the people who told you it's hard.

IN HER OWN WORDS: KAREN

Like most women, it was the myth that you need to suffer in order to get your weight under control that prevented me from escaping for all those years. I assumed it required willpower, so I always started off in a negative frame of mind. It reminded me of when I was a child and my parents would take me out for a walk. I didn't want to go because I thought it would mean slogging up and down hills and I didn't enjoy that. But they'd tell me I had no choice, so I'd stomp along in a bad mood and make every step a painful one. Because I'd decided it had to be hard, I guaranteed that it was.

Then one day we went for a walk and for some reason I found myself in a more positive frame of mind. The walking was easy and I found lots of beautiful things to enjoy along the way. It was a walk we'd taken many times before—I just hadn't allowed myself to enjoy it before.

Losing weight with Easyway reminded me of this. All it took was a change of mindset to turn it from a hard, slow, painful process to an easy and enjoyable one. And the good news is I'm still enjoying the walk. With Easyway, that happiness is forever.

A METHOD THAT WORKS

Most women assume they have two choices when it comes to losing weight: go on a diet or take a special course of exercise. Both rely on willpower because they perpetuate the myth that losing weight has to be hard. The reason everyone thinks it has to be hard is because they believe it involves some kind of sacrifice—the "giving up" of something that gives you some sort of pleasure or crutch. This couldn't be further from the truth, as you know very well.

BEING OVERWEIGHT MAKES YOU MISERABLE AND INSECURE

Throughout your life you've been bombarded with misinformation about food and drink and how certain products make you happy. It follows that the thought of having to "give up" any of your favorite foods would fill you with apprehension. The failed diets have reinforced this fear. You're caught in a no-win situation: You want to lose weight because it's making you miserable, but you're afraid that life will be miserable if you do.

But what if you were told there was a third option, an easy win, a simple method that would open that prison door without any need for willpower or hardship? What if you were given a set of instructions that promised to show you how to achieve your ideal weight easily, painlessly, and permanently, without having to diet or take up special exercise: a method that allowed you to eat as much of your favorite foods as you wanted, whenever you wanted? You would at least give it a try, wouldn't you?

You might be skeptical because you've put all your effort into opening that prison door and you're convinced that you don't have the strength, but what's your alternative? To spend the rest of your life trapped in a miserable, dark place?

When I first told people that I had found a method to cure the world of smoking, easily, painlessly, and permanently, without the need for willpower, I was greeted with skepticism. Yet tens of millions of people have succeeded in quitting smoking as a result of reading Easyway books and attending Easyway centers. And tens of thousands more turn to Easyway each year for a cure to their addiction, whether it be drugs like nicotine and alcohol, or behavioural addictions like gambling, overeating and overspending—this without ever having to rely on advertising to spread the word. Easyway has achieved worldwide success by personal recommendation, for one simple reason:

IT WORKS!

When it comes to applying a method for quitting smoking to weight loss, one obvious question leaps out. Everyone knows we can live very happily without cigarettes or other nicotine products, but we can't survive without eating. So how can a method that requires you to quit completely and permanently possibly be applied to food? I wrestled with this question too before the answer came to me from a surprising source. When it came, it was blindingly obvious.

As you begin to read this book it's only natural that all the brainwashing you've been subjected to will make you skeptical. That's fine. I realize that for anyone who has banged their head against the wall with unworkable diets and exercise regimes, the claim that there's an easy way to lose weight may seem too good to be true, or perhaps that I'm tormenting you. Rest assured, I'm doing nothing of the kind. My mission is to help you achieve the happiness that comes with freeing yourself from the weight trap.

There is no harm in questioning the Easyway claim; in fact, I positively encourage you to question everything. The reason so many people end up overweight is because they don't question what they're told.

Skepticism is perfectly understandable at this stage. It will not hamper your attempt to escape to freedom provided you don't let it stop you trying. Whatever misgivings you may have at any stage in the book, allow yourself to keep following the method and see where it takes you. There is no great effort involved. And remember the alternative: to remain trapped in a miserable prison for the rest of your life.

You don't need to change anything right now. That will all happen in good time as you reach the end of the book and, when it does, you will feel ready for it. Until then, it's important that you don't try to change your behavior or do anything that could distract you from taking in everything you read.

THE INSTRUCTIONS

You might be wondering why, if this method is so simple, you can't just skip to the end of the book and discover the secret. If that was possible, then I would encourage you to do just that. Nothing could be more convincing than leaping forward in time and seeing how you will feel when you finally free yourself from the trap you're in, but the method doesn't work like that. If you're tempted to jump ahead, you will not succeed.

There is no secret to Easyway—nothing I'm holding back for dramatic effect. It's a simple set of instructions designed to help you unravel the brainwashing that's led to your weight problem, but the instructions have to be followed in order. Think of it like the directions out of a maze or the combination lock on a safe. If I gave you a set of numbers jumbled up on a scrap of paper and you applied them in the wrong order, or you only applied some of them, the lock would remain firmly closed. Easyway is the same. It works by giving you a set of instructions that must be followed in the correct order. Follow all the instructions in order and you cannot fail to get free. That's all it takes. If at any point in the book you forget this and are tempted to skip ahead, come back to this chapter and remind yourself of the first instruction:

FIRST INSTRUCTION: FOLLOW ALL THE INSTRUCTIONS IN ORDER

By picking up this book you've already made one of the most important decisions of your life. You've picked up the key that will help you to escape the prison of being overweight. Now all you have to do is use the key. An exciting and thrilling experience lies ahead. Whatever questions you may have, whatever skepticism you may feel, they will all disappear as you read on. When you finish, you will find it hard to believe that you ever found it hard to control your weight. You will also be amazed at how good you feel and how easy it's been.

The focus of this book may be on losing weight, but the ultimate goal is your happiness. Whoever you are, whatever you do, wherever you come from, this book is the solution you've been looking for. Enjoy using it!

SUMMARY

- **Women are more susceptible to being overweight than men.**
- **Diets don't work.**
- **It's the everyday misery, not the serious health risk, that drives most attempts to lose weight.**
- **Assume it's going to be hard and you guarantee it will be.**
- **Easyway is the only method that makes it easy.**
- **First instruction: FOLLOW ALL THE INSTRUCTIONS IN ORDER.**

Chapter 2

A LESSON FROM NATURE

Why does a squirrel, when it is surrounded by an abundance of its favorite food, decide to stop eating and store up the rest for later?

In the last chapter I asked how a method for quitting smoking that requires you to quit completely and permanently can be applied to eating, and said the answer came from an unlikely source. That source was a squirrel.

Have you ever watched a squirrel eating nuts? Here's a hungry little creature, surrounded by its favorite food. What does it do, eat all of it? No, it stops after a while and stores the rest in a safe place for later. At any moment that squirrel might be startled by a predator and it will run straight up a tree as if it's the easiest feat in the world.

Imagine being that nimble and yet still being able to eat as much of your favorite food as you want. As humans, our immediate response is that the two are mutually exclusive. Any human who eats as much of their favorite food as they want tends to quickly lose the ability to move at more than walking pace, let alone run up a tree! So how come the squirrel manages to do it?

It's easy for us to see the sense in the squirrel's decision to put some nuts aside for later. As a wild animal you can never be sure where your next meal is coming from, so it's good survival practice to store food when you can. But does the squirrel really possess that level of foresight? Moreover, why don't squirrels have a weight problem? Do they know that if they overeat they won't be able to run up trees any more?

Now watch humans when a bowl of nuts is put in front of them. It's like a feeding frenzy! If members of the most intelligent species on earth are silly enough to keep gorging until the food runs out thus making themselves overweight, how come an animal with a brain the size of a nut is not so stupid? Isn't it fair to say there has to be more to it than intelligence?

It's not only squirrels that seem to be outsmarting us in this way. Think about it: Have you ever seen a wild animal of any species that was overweight? Sure, there are very fat animals like walruses and hippos, but that's the shape that nature intended them to be. It suits their lifestyle and the environment in which they live. You never see a walrus or hippo that is distinctly overweight compared to the rest of the herd.

Television has brought us some amazing images of animals in the wild and one thing that stands out is how uniform each species is in size and shape. It could be a school of fish, a herd of water buffalo, a flock of geese... their individual sizes may differ slightly, but they're all the same shape, the same proportion. There are none that lag behind the others, weighed down by an oversized belly caused by overeating.

Human intelligence isn't the only thing that sets us apart from the rest of the animal kingdom. We're also the only species on the planet that suffers with weight problems—us and the domesticated animals whose eating habits we control!

It feels like we've been left out of a secret that every other creature on the planet shares. They can eat as much of their favorite foods as they want, as often as they want to, without becoming overweight. Why can't we? Could it be that it's actually our intelligence that has been our undoing? Have we observed the animal kingdom and decided that we know better?

WHAT THEY SAY

"As long as you're feeling good with your weight and the way you look, that's what matters."
Alessandra Ambrosio, model and actress

"A cultural fixation on female thinness is not an obsession about female beauty but an obsession about female obedience."
Naomi Wolf, author

"Cook what's fresh for the day. When you're using fresh fruits, vegetables, and foods, it's easier to keep the weight

off. And I eat whatever I want—just not a ton of it."
Debi Mazar, actress

"To lose confidence in one's body is to lose confidence in oneself."
Simone De Beauvoir, philosopher

"I have high blood sugars, and Type 2 diabetes is not going to kill me. But I just have to eat right, and exercise, and lose weight, and watch what I eat, and I will be fine for the rest of my life."
Tom Hanks, actor

"I used to beat myself up about weight and working out, and no matter what I did I never felt good about myself. I decided to accept myself and know that I am good."
Ellen DeGeneres, comedian and television host

THE ROOT CAUSE

It isn't intelligence that tells the squirrel to stop eating and start storing; it's instinct. Animals don't need nutritionists or dieticians to tell them how to keep in shape; they know instinctively what they should and shouldn't eat. And so did we once upon a time. It's our intelligence that has led us to think differently, to the point where we no longer know what to think when it comes to eating.

There have been so many new diets, each one apparently

contradicting the principles of the one before. No wonder we're confused! We get bombarded with technical information and statistics that even the scientists, it seems, don't fully understand. If they did, surely one of them would have devised a diet that works by now!

In Chapter One I made the following claim:

Easyway will help you achieve your ideal weight easily, painlessly, and permanently, without having to diet or undergo special exercise, and you'll be able to eat as much of your favorite foods as you want, whenever you want.

You may have thought this sounded too good to be true—when is life ever that simple? Well, it seems fine for 99.99 percent of the animal kingdom, who all find it that simple. It has to be worth a closer look to see how they do it.

Yes, animals do struggle when food is scarce, but it's their behavior in times of abundance that is telling. Whereas humans tend to gorge themselves until they become obese, animals moderate their intake and maintain their fitness. Somehow they know when to stop.

Before we start to examine the reasons why humankind differs from the rest of the animal kingdom in this respect, it's important to deal with two possible misconceptions about my method. Firstly, it isn't magic. That is purely a figure of speech sometimes used by the happy people who have succeeded in changing their lives with this method. There is nothing complex or mysterious about the method; it's plain common sense.

Second, it's not a diet. Although we've stated that the problem is one of overeating, rather than eating, your problem is not the quantity of food you eat and the solution is not cutting down on your intake. As I will explain, overeating is a consequence of incorrect eating—essentially "junk-eating." All of this will be made perfectly clear as you read through the book. The only demand we make is that you follow all the instructions.

Still skeptical? That's perfectly normal. I've barely begun to explain the method. All we've established so far is that we, the most intelligent creatures on the planet, suffer with eating problems and being overweight while the rest of the animal kingdom does not. While they live by instinct, we use our intelligence. They eat as much of their favorite foods as they want and maintain their ideal weight without having to diet or undergo any special exercise. Clearly we have something to learn.

It's not a case of trusting this method or having faith, because it's important that you don't follow the instructions blindly. It's important that you understand the reason for each instruction; then you'll be more inclined to follow it.

SECOND INSTRUCTION: KEEP AN OPEN MIND

HOW OPEN-MINDED ARE YOU?

You may be convinced that you have an open mind, in which case the chances are it is closed. The very fact that you're convinced is a sign that you're not receptive to all possibilities. Keeping an open mind is essential for your success, so you need to be aware how easy it is to be tricked into thinking your mind is open when it's really closed.

This exercise will help. Look at the figure below. What do you see?

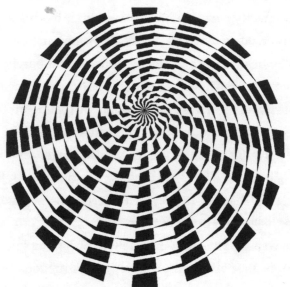

Have you made your mind up?

If you think you see a spiral, look again. It's actually a series of concentric circles. Your eyes are picking up characteristics that you associate with a spiral and your brain is jumping to the conclusion that it is a spiral. It shows how quick we are to fall back on what we've learned to be true, rather than looking at each new picture with fresh eyes and an open mind.

IN ORDER TO OPEN YOUR MIND, IT IS FIRST NECESSARY TO ACCEPT THAT IT HAS BEEN CLOSED

As you move through the book and examine the reasons why humans suffer with weight problems, you'll find yourself questioning many things about your eating habits. This can feel like a revelation. Most people never stop to question what or why they're eating: They just follow a routine laid out for them by other people, who in turn have had their routine laid out for them. When you open your mind and start asking questions, you will be amazed by the brainwashing you've been subjected to and, more importantly, you'll find it easy to unravel.

SUMMARY

- Animals eat as much of their favorite foods as they want, as often as they want but remain their ideal weight.

- The only species that has weight problems is humans (and their domesticated animals).

- The problem isn't overeating; it's incorrect eating.

- Follow the example of animals and you can achieve your ideal weight while eating as much of your favorite foods as you want, whenever you want.

- Second instruction: KEEP AN OPEN MIND.

Chapter 3

WHY YOU'RE READING THIS BOOK

IN THIS CHAPTER
•*FAVORITE FOODS* •*TASTE, OR LACK OF IT*
•*WHO CHOOSES WHAT YOU EAT?* •*THE ILLUSION OF PLEASURE*
•*WHY DIETS DON'T WORK* •*THE THIRD INSTRUCTION*

You might think you keep making bad decisions about the food you choose to eat, but are you really exercising your own free choice?

As we look more closely at the way we eat, you'll start to see why it's essential that you keep an open mind. Our approach to food is very susceptible to delusion. For example, we see lots of people who describe themselves as confirmed food lovers, yet they tell us they're not happy with their eating habits. The excitement they feel in anticipation of a meal is not matched by a sense of satisfaction afterward. Clearly there's something wrong with the way they eat, but they tell us they can't seem to change it. They keep making bad choices, which leaves them feeling weak and foolish.

They have nothing to be ashamed of because the "choices" they make when it comes to eating are not free choices at all. They're the result of a lifetime's brainwashing. When you stop and think about it, the vast majority of meals you've consumed since the day you were born were not chosen by you. You haven't been the one in control, so why should you feel guilty or ashamed about the way your eating habits have evolved?

It's also interesting that they describe themselves as "food lovers," when food leaves them feeling guilty and foolish. Evidently they love the idea of food, but the reality keeps letting them down. Therefore, it seems, they're basing their perception of themselves and their relationship with food on an illusion. This is one example of the effect of the brainwashing that we are all subjected to from birth.

The good news is that we don't have to succumb to the brainwashing and, even better, we can reverse it. It's easy. Starting right now, you're going to begin to take control of what you eat. That doesn't mean going on a diet; it means establishing a way of eating for life that leaves you satisfied and happy, just like the squirrel. We've established that you know there's something wrong with your eating habits but you can't change them. All we're doing is changing a situation that you don't like, purely so that you can enjoy life more.

YOUR FAVORITE FOODS

Achieve your ideal weight easily, painlessly, and permanently, without having to diet or undergo special exercise, while eating as much of your favorite foods as you want, whenever you want.

There are two parts to this claim that tend to cause skepticism. The first is that you can achieve your ideal weight without willpower or hardship. I will look more closely at the willpower method later in the book, by which time you will already be seeing the advantages of this one. The second part is that you can eat as much of your favourite foods as you want. You probably think you already eat as much of your favorite foods as you want and that is precisely what's given you a weight problem.

LOOK AGAIN

Remember the optical illusion in Chapter Two. What you thought was a spiral actually turned out to be a series of concentric circles. The mind can be very easily fooled, so make sure yours is open to every possibility—starting with the possibility that the foods you think are your favorites are not your favorites at all.

Let's look at what we know about these so-called favorites:
- They don't make you happy
- They don't make you feel healthy and energetic
- They make you overweight
- You wish you could find a way to eat less of them.

So what exactly is it about these foods that makes them your favorites?

Could it be the taste? That wonderful, irresistible... how would you describe it? Actually, how would you describe it? Ask anyone to describe the wonderful taste of their favorite food and you'll find they're at a loss. That's because most of the food that we tend to think of as our favorites—cookies, cakes, fries, bread, pasta etc.—actually taste bland unless they're flavored with something else.

Taste is a very suggestible sense and we confuse it with other influences, such as the setting in which we're eating or the company or the occasion. You might seem to enjoy a bottle of wine on a beachside terrace by the Mediterranean, but when you drink the same wine under a cloudy sky in England it just doesn't seem to taste as good. The power of suggestion is intense when it comes to food and drink.

Many foods that we regard as a luxury taste revolting at the first try. Oysters, caviar, foie gras, blue cheese, brandy... they all taste repugnant to anyone trying them for the first time, but because of the way they're marketed to us, we want to like them. So we persevere until we acquire the taste. What we're actually doing is becoming immune to the taste, building up a tolerance that toughens us to the foulness that made us want to retch at the first time of asking. It's not an acquired taste at all, it's

AN ACQUIRED LACK OF TASTE

Have you ever eaten a hamburger and really focused your attention on the flavors in your mouth? Now, what if someone told you the burger was made of dog meat, or rat? How do you think that would change your perception of the taste? You'd probably spit it out pretty fast. But why? What logical reason leads you to regard a cow, which spends its life covered in mud and excrement and flies, as something tasty to eat, while the thought of eating dog or rat appals you? And why is the perception reversed in other cultures, where cows are sacred and dogs are seen as food?

Is it the cow-eaters or the dog-eaters who have been brainwashed into thinking that their chosen food is the natural choice? The answer is both of them. It's clearly not the case that one meat tastes good and the other doesn't. It's the way they're presented to us that makes us decide how we perceive them to taste. Remember, your choice of food has been controlled by others from the day you were born. It's time you made your own judgment.

We're fooled into thinking the foods we consider to be our favorites are the foods that taste the best. The beautiful truth is that the foods that really taste best are, in fact, the best for you. The reason anyone finds this hard to accept is because we've been conditioned by the junk food industry into thinking the best-tasting foods are the ones we know to be bad for us.

WHY DIETS DON'T WORK FOR WOMEN

- Diets take the pleasure out of eating and eating should always be a pleasure.
- The vast majority of people who lose weight by dieting eventually put it all back on.
- Diets lead to feelings of deprivation, which can cause food disorders like binge eating.
- Your body often reacts to a diet by slowing down its metabolism, which actually makes it much harder to lose weight.

• If you feel your overeating has been caused by trauma, then diets are an obvious case of treating the symptoms rather than the cause.

• Once you've finished your diet, you go back to where you started—back to the unhealthy eating that caused weight gain in the first place. It's far better to learn healthy eating which will stand you in good stead for the rest of your life.

HOW WE'RE CONDITIONED FROM BIRTH

So if it isn't the taste that makes us choose our favorite foods, what is it? The key lies in the word "choose." The choices we make when it comes to food are not free choices at all. They've been heavily influenced since the day you were born. Were you breast-fed as a baby or given a bottle? Whose decision was that? Who decided when it was time to wean you off milk on to solids? As you grew older, did you choose the menu for school dinners, or did you "have what you were given and like it"? At work, how much choice was there in the staff canteen? And even when you came home, was it you who decided what you were having for dinner? Even if you're the one who does the cooking, you're still restricted by your budget, or perhaps your partner's tastes and what's available in the shops.

The stark fact is that most of the meals we eat from the day we're born are not the result of free choice but of conditioning by our parents and other people who have themselves been conditioned in the same way by a food industry that thrives on selling us junk.

For some people, the problem isn't the three square meals a day; it's the snacks they eat in between—the chocolate bar and package of potato chips they pick up on a whim at the checkout. This is a particular cause of guilt because it feels like free choice but it isn't. Your desire to pick up a chocolate bar will have been triggered by an association that's been fixed in your mind by conditioning, whether it's the ad campaigns of the food industry or the way your parents, grandparents or other adults used chocolate as a treat when you were a child.

The junk food marketing people aren't interested in your health and wellbeing in any way; all they're interested in is selling their product and getting as many people hooked on it as possible. There's no limit to the claims they'll make, albeit through subtle means, to create the impression that this combination of sugar and fat gives you a lift, or a degree of cool, or heightened sex appeal. Some are even sold at certain times of year only, as if they're a seasonal product like fruit!

With the false image firmly planted in your mind, all it takes is a trigger to make you think you want the chocolate bar. It could be a smell, or someone else offering it to you, or boredom, or insecurity, or habit, or desire for a reward. Whatever it is, it isn't free choice; it's conditioning.

We're also conditioned in the amount we eat. "Eat up, there are children starving in Africa." We're brought up to think it's morally wrong and impolite to leave any food behind on the plate, regardless of how much food was put on the plate in the first place. Who actually makes that decision? And if it's you, don't you tend to put more on the plate than you might consider sufficient because you don't wish to appear mean?

We've completely lost sight of how much is sufficient: Christmas dinner being the prime example. Even people who eat a moderate amount every other day of the year suddenly find themselves with a plate piled high with at least two kinds of meat and upwards of five different types of vegetables, not to mention various sauces, and they feel compelled to devour all of it. It's not surprising that most of us spend Christmas Day feeling lethargic and bloated. We've been conditioned to regard a large plateful of food as a source of happiness.

THE ILLUSION OF PLEASURE

When you tuck into that plateful of food or take the first bite of that chocolate bar, you do experience a feeling of pleasure. You attribute this pleasure to the food reinforcing the perception that it's a favorite. But if it was a genuine pleasure it would last. The pleasure of Christmas dinner often turns to pain, sometimes before you've even polished off your plateful, and that first bite of chocolate is never matched by the second, third, or fourth. What you're actually experiencing is not genuine pleasure but the illusion of pleasure that you get when you relieve a craving.

If you've ever spent a day in tight shoes, you'll know the wave of relief that washes over you when you take them off. That feels like a pleasure, but would you deliberately wear tight shoes all day just to get that feeling? When you're hooked on junk food, that's effectively what you're doing.

YOU SEEK PLEASURE IN THE VERY THING THAT'S CAUSING THE DISCOMFORT

The physical discomfort you feel when you're hungry is actually very slight. If your mind was occupied, you wouldn't even notice it. That's why your food cravings seem more intense when you're bored. The slight physical feeling triggers a response in your brain, "I need food." People who are not hooked on junk food can happily live with this until they're ready for their next meal. Indeed, the longer you wait before satisfying your hunger, the better the food will taste. That's one of the marvels of nature that I will come on to later.

When you're hooked on junk food, however, the feeling of "I need food" triggers panic. And the longer you have to wait, the greater the panic becomes. It's exactly the same process with smokers. The physical craving they feel as the nicotine from the last cigarette leaves their body is so slight as to be almost imperceptible. I call this the Little Monster.

The cries of this monster are enough to awaken a Big Monster, which lives in the brain and interprets them as "I need a cigarette". Of course, if you smoke another cigarette you merely perpetuate the cycle, but the addicted mind can't see that. It thinks the only thing that is going to relieve the craving is a cigarette and it won't be happy until it gets one.

This is how addiction works. Ask a smoker what appeals to them about cigarettes and they might tell you they like the taste. In fact, they're not aware of the taste when they smoke. What they're feeling is the relief from the craving for their nicotine fix.

Now you should be able to see how that applies to eating: What you tell yourself is a delicious sensory experience is actually just the relief of getting your fix.

You might crave Christmas lunch or other favorite foods because you associate them with happy occasions. It's just another case of conditioning. When you analyze any happy occasion that you associate with food, you find that it would have been happy with or without the food. Christmas, a birthday, a date, a holiday—remember that bottle of wine. Take away the food and the occasion is still happy. Take away the occasion and the food just isn't the same.

ADDICTION

I called my method Easyway because originally it provided smokers with an easy way to quit smoking. The same method has worked successfully for people with other addictions, including alcohol and other drugs as well as gambling. Perhaps you balk at the suggestion that junk eating is an addiction. It really doesn't matter what label you put on it; the fact is that many of the products that are peddled to us by the food and drink industry get us hooked in the same way that smokers get hooked on nicotine. Don't be put off if I refer to it as an addiction. You'll come to see that it's actually helpful to view the problem in those terms.

A POSITIVE MINDSET

It's the fear of sacrificing a pleasure that makes people miserable at the prospect of losing weight. With Easyway, there is no need to feel miserable about what's in prospect. On the contrary, you have so much to look forward to. The only reason you might feel despondent when you first read the claim is because you remember the misery you've been through trying to diet. You've been brainwashed into thinking losing weight is hard and the fact that the diet didn't solve your weight problem makes you feel like you weren't up to it. Get it clear in your mind: Any diet that's failed you in the past didn't fail because you weren't strong enough; it failed because it was asking the impossible: to spend the rest of your life feeling like you're making a sacrifice, while remaining happy with the way you eat. It's a contradiction that is doomed to failure.

You might point to other people for whom a diet does appear to have worked. You hold yourself up against these people and feel inadequate, a failure. But look more closely. Most diets bring some success to begin with. Of course they do: They generally involve reducing the amount you consume, which, assuming you continue to move about to the same degree, will inevitably lead to a loss in weight. But it doesn't last.

As soon as you come off the diet, the weight piles back on again.

The only thing a diet achieves is to make food appear more precious. It provides no long-term plan, so when you finally reach your target weight, what happens next? Do you stick to the diet? Well, no, of course not. You're happy with the weight you are and you don't want to keep eating that miserable ration they put you on. So you abandon the diet and you probably treat yourself to a little reward. In a fraction of the time it took you to lose the weight, you've put it all back on and more.

The few people who appear to succeed in keeping their weight down long term through dieting are usually those for whom it's absolutely essential: models, actresses, dancers, jockeys, boxers, athletes. For them, the need to keep to a certain weight gives them an extra reason to resist the temptation to eat. But don't be fooled into thinking they've succeeded and you've failed. They don't find it easy and they don't find it enjoyable. It's the sacrifice they make for their profession and when their career ends and they no longer have to restrict themselves, they often balloon in size.

Don't regard these people as dietary successes. Success is achieving your ideal weight with ease—while being perfectly happy with the food that you eat.

AND BEING HAPPY!

As long as you feel you're making a sacrifice, you will never succeed in solving a weight problem. The same applies to smoking and all other addictions. If you continue to be taken in by the illusion of pleasure, you will always feel deprived if you have to go without your little crutch. The longer you have to go without it, the more precious it will become.

You're reading this book for the purely selfish reason that you want to feel better about yourself and enjoy eating without feeling guilty and miserable afterward. That's a brilliant aim.

YOU CAN'T ACHIEVE HAPPINESS IF YOU FEEL DEPRIVED

It's time to stop focusing on what you think you might miss out on and focus instead on everything you stand to gain. You're not being asked to "give up" anything; you're being shown how to rid yourself of a monster that's making you miserable, threatening your health, wasting your money, and leaving you feeling weak and pathetic. In its place you're gaining in fitness, energy, health, and happiness, and without food being the obsession that it has been you'll find you have more time too for all the genuine pleasures in life.

So discard any feelings of despondency. This is an exciting time. Your decision to pick up this book and do something positive about your weight is one of the best decisions you've ever made. You're not just going to lose weight; you're going to gain an understanding of your body and the way you eat that is as natural and easy as a squirrel scaling a tree. So rejoice! All you have to do is keep your mind open and keep following the instructions.

THIRD INSTRUCTION: START OFF WITH A FEELING OF ELATION!

SUMMARY

- Think again about the foods that you enjoy most. If they made you happy, you wouldn't be reading this book.

- Next time you eat one of your favorite foods, focus on the taste. Is it really that great?

- Your taste has been heavily influenced by conditioning; it's time to free yourself and make your own choices.

- The pleasure you think you get from junk is just an illusion. It doesn't last.

- Diets do nothing but make food seem more precious.

- There's no need to mope.

- Third instruction: START OFF WITH A FEELING OF ELATION!

Chapter 4

THE TRAP

IN THIS CHAPTER
• *THREE MYTHS* • *A TUG-OF-WAR*
• *WHY YOU THINK IT'S HARD* • *EXCUSES*
• *WHAT YOU STAND TO GAIN*

You don't overeat because you're weak; you overeat because you're caught in a fiendish trap. Understand the trap and escape not only becomes possible; it becomes easy.

You might not have thought of your weight problem as a trap before, but that's exactly what it is. You're lured in by the promise of something marvelous. Like everyone else in the world, you've been brainwashed to believe that junk food gives you some sort of pleasure or crutch.

The pleasure is nothing more than an illusion, but you don't know that—no one tells you that, not even the medical experts who spend their lives trying to tackle obesity. All the information you have is that these foods are hard to resist, so you continue to seek that unknown pleasure.

Rather than coming to the logical conclusion that the pleasure doesn't exist, you assume you're not getting enough, so you increase your intake.

HOW THE TRAP WORKS

You've probably come across the pitcher plant, that carnivorous funnel-shaped trap that lures flies into its digestive chamber with the sweet smell of nectar. The fly lands on the rim and begins to feed. The nectar seems like the best thing in the world, but it's luring the fly to its death. As it feeds, the fly slips unwittingly further and further toward the chamber until it falls right in and the plant consumes it.

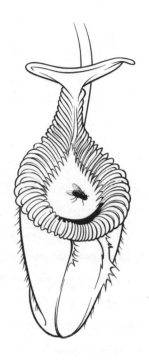

The addiction trap works in a very similar way. The difference between junk addiction and other addictions is that we land on the rim of the pitcher plant before we are old enough to realize what we are doing. By the time we develop some awareness of the nutritional value of the foods we eat, we are well on our way down the slippery slope.

Yet we see millions of other people doing the same, many of them with no apparent ill effects at all, and at the same time we are bombarded with false information about how these foods will make us happy, cool, sexy... So we close our eyes and carry on consuming. Like the fly, we slip further and further down the slope. We think we're eating what we want to eat out of choice, but the truth is that before we're even aware of what is good for us and what is not, **WE'VE ALREADY LOST CONTROL!**

The trap works like a noose that tightens the more you pull on it. The harder you try to escape, the more trapped you become. It's a fiendish trick of the mind that makes you do the opposite of what's good for you.

YOU SEEK RELIEF IN THE VERY THING THAT'S MAKING YOU MISERABLE

This is exactly how addiction takes hold. It is 1 percent physical and 99 percent mental. The drug doesn't give you a high. On the contrary, it makes you feel below par as it leaves your system, but instead of accepting that the drug does nothing for you, the Big Monster in your brain, which was created by all the brainwashing, convinces you that it's the one thing that can pick you up again. It quickly becomes a vicious circle: Every time you turn to the drug for relief, you start the next round of craving.

The food you eat has hooked you in exactly the same way. As long as you go on believing that it's the one thing that can give you pleasure or a crutch, you'll remain in the trap and your attempts to lose weight will always end in failure.

But the opposite is also true: Once you can see that junk food does absolutely nothing for you whatsoever, it becomes obvious that the only way to feel back on par is to stop eating it.

Instead of pulling on the noose, relax and unravel the knot. When you no longer regard junk as a pleasure or crutch, the desire for it goes and stopping becomes easy. All you have to do is reverse the brainwashing.

> **JUNK**
>
> Later in the book I will go into more detail about the food and drink that hooks you like a drug and prevents you from losing weight. For the sake of simplicity, I'll refer to all such food and drink as "junk" or "junk food." This covers any food or drink that contributes to your weight problem.

THE VOID

There are three key pieces of brainwashing that lead us into the trap in the first place:

- The myth that the human mind and body are weak and need outside help in order to enjoy life and cope with stress
- The myth that junk will compensate for these illusory weaknesses
- The myth that humans are more intelligent than the intelligence that created us, whatever you believe that to be.

From the day we're born we seek comfort and security from those around us. If we're lucky, it's provided by loving parents, but as we grow older we begin to see through their veneer of indestructibility and our insecurities resurface. At the same time we're thrown into unfamiliar environments that can be bewildering—new schools, clubs and workplaces—and we feel an unnerving sense of emptiness, a void that we try to fill with pop stars, movie stars, and other fantasy role models. Our dependence on these role models for our sense of self makes us very susceptible to negative influences. If our heroes smoke, we're likely to smoke. If they drink, we drink. And if they eat junk, we eat junk.

Remember, all our role models have gone through the same search for reassurance and they've all been brainwashed just as we have.

The void creates the belief that we, as a species, are weak and incomplete, which in turn creates our desire for something to fill the gap. The illusion that junk compensates for our weakness makes us dependent on it. It's a classic con trick, like selling a crutch riddled with woodworm to someone who doesn't have a broken leg.

THE BELIEF THAT WE ARE WEAK AND INCOMPLETE INSURES THAT WE REMAIN WEAK AND INCOMPLETE

It's a self-fulfilling con, sold to us by people with a vested interest in keeping us hooked on junk.

THE DIFFERENT TYPES OF EATING

How often do you eat simply because you're physically hungry: for example when you have low blood sugar? It can be a very useful exercise to reflect on why exactly you eat what you eat in the way that you do.

SOCIAL EATING—everyday eating with your family, or on special occasions such as birthdays and weddings, or meals with friends

EMOTIONAL EATING—this includes comfort eating (when you are feeling miserable or tired and cold—comfort eating may feel good at the time but often feeds a cycle of guilt or leads to binge eating), snacking to combat stress and boredom, or as compensation for when you're feeling upset or rushed off your feet

IMPULSE EATING—you walk past a bakery and smell baking bread, or see a selection of cakes in the window. Or you might see an advert on television. Your appetites are deliberately stimulated all the time.

There are many external cues which will make you feel hungry—experts say that we make around 220 "eating decisions" every day. Emotional eating is more common in women than in men, but given the choice men are also more likely to opt for larger portions.

A MENTAL TUG-OF-WAR

One of the great frustrations of being overweight is that even when we wake up to the fact that the way we eat is making us miserable we feel powerless to stop. It's a sort of schizophrenia: The rational part of your brain will tell you that your eating is putting you at risk of serious health problems, wasting your money, and making you despise yourself and that the logical thing to do is stop, yet the subconscious part continues to harbor a desire to eat. The reason your subconscious mind doesn't follow the logic of your rational mind is because it's been conditioned to believe a different "truth": that the food you eat gives you some sort of pleasure or crutch.

Unfortunately, the subconscious mind is a much stronger influence over your behavior than the rational mind. It governs happiness and the pursuit of happiness is ultimately what governs all our actions. Happiness is the emotion we feel when we satisfy hunger and thirst, or find security and love.

These are the base instincts that insure the survival of our species, and desire for happiness is the emotion that drives us to pursue them. So whatever we believe makes us happy is the path we will pursue.

Throughout your life you've been told that certain food and drink gives you pleasure or a crutch. Everywhere you look there are images of smiling, happy people devouring junk. Yet in your rational mind you've lost sight of any pleasure. No matter how hard you try to let the rational side lift you out of the trap, the emotional side keeps dragging you back in.

What you want to do is regain control and let your rational mind win the day. You can't do that through willpower because that will only make your emotional side feel more deprived. In order to win the tug-of-war you must undo the brainwashing that has created the desire to eat junk.

This is easier than you might think, but first you have to

recognize and accept that you have been brainwashed and take a positive attitude to undoing it. It sounds simple, but this is the part that overeaters find incredibly hard and that's why they end up failing to escape from the trap.

As we said in Chapter One, it's the belief that getting free will be hard that makes it hard. The difference between Easyway and all the other methods that claim to help overcome addiction is that the other methods begin with the message that it will not be easy. This alone is another piece of brainwashing that unwittingly keeps addicts in the trap because,

THE HARDER YOU THINK QUITTING IS GOING TO BE, THE MORE FEARFUL YOU WILL BE OF TRYING

So let's look more closely at why you might think it will be hard.

FAILURES

Presumably you know plenty of people who have tried to lose weight through dieting or exercise or a combination of the two but have always ended up piling the pounds back on again. They might succeed for a month, a year, or even several years, but if they end up overweight again then the diet has failed, hasn't it? All diets fail in the end because they don't make you happy. The only way to maintain your ideal weight for life is to make sure you genuinely enjoy mealtimes and don't feel deprived.

You may question this. There are lots of overweight people who appear to enjoy mealtimes and don't feel deprived. They don't bother dieting because they don't care about being fat.

Really? Do you honestly believe that? If you care about being overweight, why do you think they don't? You know the misery it causes: the physical discomfort, the lethargy, the sense of helplessness. Do you honestly think there are people who enjoy feeling that way? Isn't it more likely that they conceal their misery behind a mask—the jovial glutton—and would jump at the chance to be their ideal weight if only they could?

They will have tried to diet and failed. Every failed diet is a major setback. They see their failure as a reflection of themselves and regard themselves as pathetic, weak, and inferior to all those people who appear to sail through life without such problems. At the same time, they reinforce their belief that being overweight is an impregnable prison from which they'll never have the strength to escape. And when they look at all the other failed dieters, it only serves to strengthen this belief further still.

When you look at these examples, and even when you look at yourself, you see people who are, in many ways, strong. Overeaters aren't all weak, foolish people. On the contrary, many of the world's most intelligent, strong-minded people have been overweight. It's not because they want to be overweight, nor is it because losing weight is harder than running a country or a big business, say. It's simply because they've gone about it the wrong way.

If you tried to open a can of soup with a corkscrew, would you blame your lack of willpower when it didn't work?

IT'S WHO I AM

Another factor that puts people off trying to lose weight is the belief that they'll lose a valuable part of their identity. Despite the misery, the slavery, the ill health, the torment, the loss of self-respect, and all the other damaging effects caused by junk eating, some people will continue to see their problem as something that makes them the person they are. They feel it's their duty to be the one who consumes up the last crumbs of cake or drinks the last drop of wine. It just shows how the trap can twist your judgment.

These poor people are under the illusion that overeating makes them more loveable. In popular entertainment, as in life, we tend to feel intimidated by characters who show no vulnerability and we warm to the ones who are flawed. The tragic character who battles through life against her own demons, be it food, drink, drugs or whatever, usually wins our sympathy and affection over the one who appears to be in complete control and never puts a foot out of place. We're bombarded with these stereotypes over and over again so it's no wonder that our own self-image often appears more attractive if there are obvious flaws. We worry that if we take the eating problem out of our life, we'll take on the attributes of the intimidating, invulnerable character and lose what we perceive to be our "charm."

Get it clear in your mind: There is nothing charming or loveable about being a glutton. Obesity is not charming, nor are diabetes, high blood pressure, heart disease, strokes, or cancer. So if you're being held back by a belief that you'll lose your individual place in society if you stop eating junk, you can let that thought go now.

When you quit you will be amazed how much better you feel: fitter, more confident, more relaxed. All these things will make you more attractive and engaging to those around you, but above all, you'll love yourself more.

EXCUSES

Everyone who overeats wishes they could stop. The fact that they can't makes them feel foolish and weak. It's a miserable feeling so they try to cover it up by inventing excuses for why they continue to overeat.

"It's just the way I'm made."

"I love my food."

"It comforts me."

"I just do it to be sociable."

"I don't have time to eat healthily."

These excuses are just delusions. They imply that you make a controlled decision over everything you eat, but as everyone who is struggling with an eating problem knows,

YOU DON'T CONTROL JUNK FOOD;
IT CONTROLS YOU

It's not easy to admit this. When you're in the trap, it seems far easier to bury your head in the sand and deny that you have a problem. Admitting that you have a problem forces you to face your options, which are:

• Stay in the trap and continue to suffer the misery

OR

• Get out.

Getting out is more intimidating than staying in because you've been brainwashed into believing it will be painful and that you will spend the rest of your life feeling deprived. Faced with that prospect, the familiarity of the trap seems the lesser of two evils.

But making excuses just so you don't have to face up to your problem is not going to save you from harm. As we all know, the ostrich that buries its head in the sand is all the more vulnerable for doing so.

The good news is that getting out of the trap doesn't have to be painful or difficult. Once you can see that and visualize all the wonderful benefits that come with getting free, the choice becomes easy.

THE EASY OPTION

I began this book by detailing the damaging consequences of being overweight. These consequences should not be ignored, but my aim is not to scare you into quitting. If shock tactics worked, I wouldn't hesitate to use them but they don't. It's much more effective to focus on the benefits that await you when you quit.

Health and fitness

When you're free of junk, you'll find that you suffer fewer illnesses and recover more quickly when you do fall ill. You'll be happier with what you see in the mirror, which will give you a greater feeling of wellbeing overall. You'll have more energy and will be less susceptible to stress and anxiety. You'll feel aglow with health and happiness.

Control

Regaining control over your eating also enables you to control other aspects of your life better. You'll feel life is less frenetic and you'll be able to make plans that will leave you feeling happy and fulfilled.

Honesty

Free from the need for excuses and denial, you'll no longer feel the need to cover your tracks. Dishonesty causes stress, shame and anger.

When you can look at yourself in the mirror without shame, it will feel like a weight being lifted from your shoulders.

Self-respect

The realization that you're no longer a slave to junk will make you feel much better about yourself. Every time you think about your achievement in escaping the trap, you'll feel a burst of elation and pride. Feeling great about how you look is priceless.

Time

It's hard to find time for everything in life when eating is your preoccupation. You might think you eat junk now because you don't have time to cook proper meals, but, in fact, that's an illusion that you will see through when you're free.

Money

The more junk you eat, the more you spend. The belief that healthy eating costs more is another myth, which we will explode later in the book. When you're not constantly hungry, you will save a fortune on snacks and other junk foods that give you nothing of nutritional value.

SUMMARY

- **The trap makes you do the opposite of what's good for you.**
- **Accept that escape can be easy and it will be.**
- **Nobody is happy being overweight.**
- **If people find you sexy and fun, it's despite your weight problem, not because of it.**
- **You have everything to gain and nothing to lose.**

Chapter 5

THE INCREDIBLE MACHINE

The human body has everything it needs to survive and thrive without external influences. All you need are the instructions that make it tick.

Have you ever bought a new car? If not, no doubt you know someone who has. It becomes the most precious thing in their life. They wince at the thought of any harm coming to it. The slightest scratch has them peering with concern. They'll wash it, polish it, furnish it with fancy features. And why not? The car is a truly remarkable machine. But you have in your possession a far more incredible machine than a car:

THE HUMAN BODY

It can perform millions of functions all at the same time without you even realizing. What's more, you can scratch it or even break it and it will repair itself. It needs no outside help. Your body's ability to recover from the abuse you put it through is so remarkable it puts any manufactured machine to shame.

The notion that the human mind and body are weak is a myth. So is the belief that we need outside help to compensate for any weakness. The human body is capable of producing every drug and every instinctive reaction it needs to survive. It produces antibodies that fight disease and build a protective barrier against future infection, and it boasts an early warning system—pain—designed to send you a clear signal when something is wrong. Pain is a crucial function in our built-in survival mechanism. It's like the oil warning light in a car. It tells us there's a problem and, if we've got any sense, we deal with the problem.

Our senses are also part of that early warning system. Sight, smell, hearing, touch, and taste all play a vital role in keeping us alive. Watch an animal when it approaches food. It doesn't have to be a wild animal; domesticated cats will give a perfectly good demonstration. Watch them out in the open. If there's food about they won't go straight up to it: They'll look around, sniff the air, and cock their ears for any hint of danger. Only when they're satisfied that they're not about to be pounced on themselves will they approach the food, always looking around, sniffing and listening. When they get to the food they won't just tuck in. First they'll look at it from a safe distance, then they'll go up and sniff it. They might prod it with a paw, and then, if all these senses are satisfied, they'll taste it, tentatively at first. They're using their senses to detect danger from their environment and from the food. If it's poison, they will spot it, smell it, feel it, or taste it well before they ever swallow it.

Believe it or not, your senses do the same for you. You can tell when an apple is rotten just by looking at it. If it's just on the turn it might look edible, but it will smell off and will be soft to the touch.

If you took a bite, the taste would be repugnant and you would spit it out. An experience like that might put you off apples for a while. There are no role models or friends pressurizing you to persevere.

We're brainwashed into consuming all manner of poisons: coffee, alcohol, nicotine, moldy cheese… Your first reaction is revulsion when you're introduced to these poisons. Your senses are trying to protect you. Poisons might be designed to look appealing, but the smell is your first warning. The taste is your second. That first taste of alcohol makes a lot of people gag. If you manage to get enough of it down, the chances are you'll be sick. This is the next line of defense as your body does everything it can to expel the poison.

The human body is incredible in its natural defense against things that are bad for us. Put the wrong fuel in your car, on the other hand, and the first you'll know about it is when the engine grinds to a halt. Why then, with all these protective systems in place, do we find it so hard to keep ourselves in peak working condition?

THE FLAW IN THE INCREDIBLE MACHINE

Your body's resilience makes it infinitely more incredible than any machine ever invented by humankind, yet it is also your undoing. It's all too easy to take your body for granted: abuse it one day, recover the next. Wild animals have the same powers of recovery, yet you don't see them abusing their bodies in the way humans do. This is down to the one fundamental difference between humans and the rest of the animal kingdom:

INTELLECT

We have the same instinctive capacity for survival as other animals, but we also have the intellectual capacity to disregard our instincts. Somewhere in our evolution intellect has gained the upper hand.

Our intellect has given us the capacity to learn and pass on our learning. As a result, we've developed into a highly sophisticated species that is not only capable of building fantastic structures and machines but also has an appreciation of art, music, romance, spirituality, and so on. Intellect is a wonderful thing, but it can go to your head. We consider ourselves above other animals and in many ways we are, but when it comes to eating properly and staying fit, we have a lot to learn.

The flaw in the incredible machine is that we trust our intellect above our instincts. We consider instinct to be animalistic, whereas intellect is sophisticated. But look again at the "advances" humankind has made and you'll see that, rather than building on the advantage that Mother Nature has given us, we've devoted a remarkable amount of intellect to self-destruction. By allowing our intellect to override our instincts, we've become a species of compulsive junk consumers.

NATURE'S WARNING LIGHT

When the oil light comes on in your car, you have three options:

- Ignore it
- Remove the bulb
- Top up the engine oil.

Only one thing will prevent the engine from seizing up.

Pain is nature's warning light and stupidly we tend to treat it the same way. We either ignore it until it becomes intolerable, by which time the problem has become severe, possibly even life-threatening, or we take painkillers. This is the same principle as removing the bulb. All it does is remove the symptom, not the cause. Yet we regard the pharmaceutical industry as one of the great triumphs of human intellect, when all it has done is override our natural ability to protect ourselves from injury and disease.

If you regularly take medication for indigestion, you're merely removing the bulb from the warning light. Wouldn't you rather remove whatever's causing the indigestion?

ONE SIDE OF THE STORY

Because we no longer live by our instincts in the way that animals do, we tend to regard them as hit or miss—nothing more than guesswork. But instinct is not hit or miss; it is the result of millions of years of trial and error. It's what enables every creature on Earth to find their own favorite food without eating anything that harms them. It also enables them to breed with far less trouble than humans. Wild animals don't need books and learning to keep reproducing. Instinct is their guide.

It is our tendency to trust in intellectual opinion over and above our own instincts; that is the flaw that leads us into the junk trap. When we make intellectual choices based on misinformation—like eating cake for comfort, for example—our wellbeing suffers. Wild animals don't get overweight or experience bouts of guilt after they've eaten. Only humans do. Intellect causes misery just as it causes happiness. The choice is ours, so why do we so often take the self-destructive option? Quite simply,

WE DON'T ALWAYS REALIZE WE HAVE AN OPTION

Has anybody ever told you cake is virtually tasteless without additives, as are chips, chocolate, cookies, cheese, meat, pasta, potatoes, and just about every other food we commonly regard as our favorites? Or is this the first time that thought has crossed your mind? When you spend your life being bombarded with images of people apparently getting huge pleasure from eating these things, it's the natural intellectual response to believe what they're telling you.

The trouble is there are plenty of people who stand to gain from keeping you in the dark. Drug companies, the tobacco and alcoholic drinks industries, the food industry, gambling firms... they've all become expert at exploiting our intellect to hoodwink us into making misguided choices.

Nobody chooses to be overweight. We don't start eating junk thinking, "Great! I'm on my way to becoming obese!" We eat it because we think it gives us some sort of pleasure or crutch. Our instincts may be screaming at us to stop, doing everything in their power to reject the poison, but we push through the pain barrier because we believe it's worth it.

It's time to open your mind to the possibility that everything you've ever been told about the food you eat is untrue. Put your preconceptions to one side and start judging the facts for yourself. Imagine if you could convince yourself of one fundamental fact:

EATING JUNK DOES ABSOLUTELY NOTHING FOR YOU WHATSOEVER

Wouldn't that make it easy to stop?

SWEET NOTHING

Fruit and vegetables are the food that nature designed us to eat above any other and our taste for the natural sugar in fruit is designed to keep us coming back for more. Refined sugar, packed into junk food and alcoholic drinks, is manufactured to replicate the sweetness of fruit. It contains none of the goodness of fruit, but it tricks our taste buds into thinking it's the same thing. That's why we regard so many sugar-packed foods as our favourites; when we eat them we feel a boost while our craving for sugar is temporarily satisfied. It's the illusion of pleasure. Intellectually, we've created a substance that fools our instincts into thinking we're getting something good when, in truth, it's nothing but bad.

TRUTH OR ILLUSION?

Your desire for junk comes from the belief that it gives you some sort of pleasure or crutch. At the same time the fear of living without it makes it hard for you to "give it up." You've reached this point in your life believing that certain foods are your favorites. Now I'm telling you that they do absolutely nothing for you whatsoever. How are you supposed to know what's right and how can you be completely convinced?

First of all, let's remember why you're reading this book. You want to stop eating junk and free yourself from the trap that's prevented you from becoming the weight you want to be. Will you achieve that if you decide to believe that I'm wrong and the illusion of pleasure you get from eating junk really is a genuine pleasure? Or will that just leave you exactly where you were when you made the decision to pick up this book?

Now, if you choose to go along with me and stop eating junk, what do you think will happen?

But I don't want you to go along with me out of blind faith. You have to be convinced about your decision. Fortunately, there's an easy way to clear away the doubt and be absolutely sure what is truth and what is illusion.

Think back to the spiral diagram in Chapter Two. Once you're told that it's actually a series of concentric circles, you can always see it for yourself. It might continue to look like a spiral at first glance, but all you have to do is look closely with that knowledge in mind and you'll always be able to see it as it really is.

Here's another illusion that illustrates the point. Here are some irregular black shapes. Look hard at the black shapes. Do you see a message?

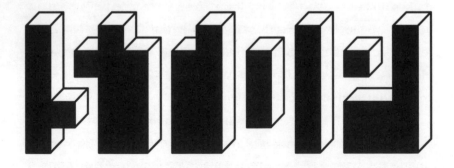

At first, it might look like a random line of building blocks. If so, look again. This time look at the shapes with your eyes half-closed (through your eyelashes) and you can make a word appear. It might help if you move your head back a little (or to one side) and look again from a distance. You should see the word "STOP."

The word hasn't suddenly appeared; it's been there all along. If you couldn't see it that's because you thought you were looking at irregular black shapes. After all, that is what you were told. So you were focusing on the black rather than the white shapes in between.

Once you can see the word "STOP," it becomes impossible to look at the pattern and not see it. But until you're told it's there, you could very well never find it. *And once you've seen the truth, you can never be fooled again.*

This illusion deliberately misleads you into looking at the blocks rather than the words, just as the food industry deliberately misleads you into believing that junk gives you some sort of pleasure or crutch.

Only Easyway points out the alternative: that junk does absolutely nothing for you whatsoever. When you start to examine this side of the argument, you quickly see that it's true and you can never again be fooled into believing the opposite.

You fell into the trap because you were under the illusion that junk gave you pleasure and/or a crutch. And yet it's not made you happy and secure, it's made you miserable and afraid. It's also left you overweight and unable to do anything about it. The truth is plain to see and now that you've seen it, nothing will be able to change your perception.

EATING FOR TWO

According to the European Association for the Study of Diabetes, it isn't a good idea at all for women to "eat for two" during pregnancy. It's best for women to be in "optimal health at a healthy weight and to maintain this during and after pregnancy." Women who are obese before pregnancy (with a BMI of 30 or higher) and who gain excess weight are 43 times more likely to develop Type 2 diabetes.

Nor is dieting a good option for expectant mothers—it can lead to premature birth and underweight babies—but overeating the wrong foods is also damaging.

In fact, pregnancy is the perfect time to eat a nutritious and balanced diet.

MOTHER NATURE'S GUIDE

The reason we regard childbirth as a miracle is because the reproduction of life is way beyond the capacity of our intelligence. The object of this chapter has been to show you that, no matter how great have been the achievements of humankind, they pale into insignificance next to the achievements of Mother Nature.

We've established that your body is in fact infinitely more sophisticated and powerful than any machine designed by humankind, but manufactured machines are easy to maintain because they come with a user guide written by the manufacturer —the leading authority on how that machine works.

Whatever your belief may be about how human beings came into existence, we can agree on one thing: we weren't designed by a human. Therefore, humankind is not the leading authority on how the body works. There is a higher authority that created us, whether you believe that to be God, evolution, or whatever.

For the sake of argument, let's refer to our maker as Mother Nature. She did an incredible job when she designed the human being. If only she'd provided us with a manufacturer's guide to tell us how best to look after ourselves, then we wouldn't have to rely on the opinion of doctors, nutritionists, and other so-called experts who keep changing their theories about what we should and shouldn't eat.

GOOD NEWS—SHE DID!

All living creatures are born with their own manufacturer's guide. It's how our ancestors survived long before the supermarket, the ready meal, the microwave, and the nutritionist came on the scene. They didn't need to be told about calories and vitamins, any more than you need to be told about the workings of the internal combustion engine for you to keep your car running. They simply followed Mother Nature's Guide.

That's how wild animals continue to survive without becoming overweight. They're much more selective than us about the food they eat and they don't suffer from constipation, diarrhea, heartburn, indigestion, stomach ulcers, irritable bowel syndrome, high blood pressure, high cholesterol, and diseases of the stomach, bowel, kidneys, and liver.

Nor do they die from strokes, diabetes, cancer or heart disease. These conditions are the direct result of our eating habits, which have become established as a result of following our intellect rather than Mother Nature's Guide.

Before we look more closely at the instructions that we were intended to follow by Mother Nature, we need to decide on our ultimate objective: your ideal weight.

SUMMARY

- **The human body and mind are incredibly strong and do not need outside help.**

- **Junk can't compensate for any human weakness, illusory or otherwise.**

- **Trusting our intellect over our instinct has brought us untold misery.**

- **Once you see both sides of an argument, you can choose which one to believe. If you only see one side, you're being brainwashed.**

- **The leading authority on how your body works is Mother Nature.**

Chapter 6

ESTABLISHING YOUR IDEAL WEIGHT

IN THIS CHAPTER
A TARGET WEIGHT *YOU CAN'T FOOL YOUR EYES*
THE FOURTH INSTRUCTION
ONE THIRD OF YOUR PROBLEM SOLVED

How will you know when you've achieved your ideal weight? And how will you feel along the way?

There are three aspects to the problem of weight control that can make it hard to keep sight of what you're trying to achieve. They are:

• How to work out your ideal weight
• How to dispose of weight
• How to control your intake.

When we talk about your ideal weight, you probably have a figure in mind. Such is the obsession with diets and exercise these days that most of us will have been told the weight we should be for our height. There's no shortage of sources that will give you this information and we tend to carry it with us, like an ID card, always there to remind us, "This is the weight you should be."

Well, now you can throw that little reminder away. It's useless to you. In fact, it's a hindrance for three reasons:

• It's inaccurate

• It damages your self-esteem

• It disregards Mother Nature's Guide.

Weight charts are the product of an inexact science. There are many factors that contribute to your weight and these differ for each individual. Bone size, for example. Don't be taken in by the liberal use of scientific jargon that's scattered around these weight charts; it's totally unscientific to suggest that there is a simple equation revolving around height and weight that applies to everybody.

Because they are notoriously unscientific, weight charts provide a convenient excuse for the unsuccessful weight-watcher. When you fail to hit that target you can say, "Oh well, those charts aren't accurate anyway." What's the point in setting a target that you don't wholeheartedly believe in? All it does is guarantee failure.

GUESS THE WEIGHT

An exercise that always gets interesting results in the group sessions at my lose-weight centers is when I ask attendees to consider a famous athlete and guess how much they weigh. I generally go for the fastest man on Earth, but why not choose Jessica Ennis-Hill, world and

Olympic heptathlon champion. What do you think Ennis-Hill weighs?

What makes this exercise interesting is that estimates usually vary by many, many pounds. There'll be some debate in the room, some scratching of heads, and then they'll say, "Come on then, what's the answer?" At this point I have to disappoint them. I have absolutely no idea how much Jessica Ennis-Hill weighs. I don't need to. The point, which we're all agreed on, is that she's in superb physical condition. We don't need a set of scales to know that. If you were in similar physical shape, do you think you'd care how much you weighed?

The fact that estimates of another person's weight can vary by many, many pounds shows that we actually have no idea about the correlation between what the scales tell us and what we see when we look in the mirror. Think about your own case. Did you decide it was time to lose weight when the scales went over a certain figure, or was it the sight of your reflection in the mirror, the fact that your clothes started to feel too tight, you felt sluggish, and got out of breath at the slightest exertion?

If you set yourself a target weight, you won't feel that you've achieved anything until the scales show that you've hit that weight. It could take weeks; it could take years.

In the meantime, you'll feel that you're suffering as you wait for the moment of fulfilment and you'll become increasingly disappointed with yourself as the days slide by.

A target weight is supposed to be a carrot to incentivize you toward your goal, but it is actually a stick to beat yourself with until you get there. And if you do ever arrive, what happens if you look at the scales one day and see that you've gained a pound? Even though by then you may be many, many pounds lighter than you are now, that single pound can make you feel just as miserable.

So forget about mathematics or guesswork. They are as much use to you as they are to the rest of the animal kingdom. Squirrels maintain their ideal weight without any concept of what weight is! Remember, simplicity is the guiding principle of Easyway, so let's not complicate it with calculations.

FOURTH INSTRUCTION: DISPENSE WITH ANY TARGET WEIGHT

FEELING FINE

It's not your scales that will tell you when you're the exact weight you want to be; it's your eyes and your lungs. When you can look at yourself full-length in the mirror, wearing only your underwear, and admire what you see; when you wake up every morning bursting with energy and looking forward to each new day with confidence and joy—that's when you'll know you've achieved your ideal weight.

Waking up full of energy, admiring your reflection in the

mirror, feeling confident and excited about the new day: these are feelings we associate with being young but tend to give up on as we grow older. We assume that ageing brings a loss of energy and strength and a greater sense of pressure, of stress, of time running out, and so we relinquish the unbridled joy of youth all too easily.

The fact of the matter is that the feelings we put down to ageing are largely caused by our poor diet. When you start eating according to Mother Nature's Guide and stop being a slave to junk, your energy and strength come flooding back and you find the pressures of life become easier to handle. The happiness that you thought was a thing of the past returns and you can feel like you're living life to the full once more.

This is a wonderful feeling and it's one that we're all designed to achieve. There may be aspects of your physical appearance, other than your weight, that you wish were different: a smaller nose perhaps, or bigger eyes. Easyway can't do anything about that, but I can promise you that as you get closer to your ideal weight, such details will bother you less and less. We all tend to be our own harshest critics. As your inner happiness increases, you'll begin to see yourself as other people see you: radiating health, confidence, and happiness. Those are the most attractive features in any person. This in turn will give your inner happiness an extra boost, and so the good feeling will become self-perpetuating.

It's the opposite to the vicious circle you find yourself in when you're not happy with your weight. You radiate unhappiness, which in turn makes you less outwardly attractive, which makes you more unhappy. Doesn't it feel great to be putting a stop to that destructive cycle?

DON'T THROW AWAY THE SCALES

Hopefully, you're reading this carefully and will have noticed that I said the cycle of happiness will kick in "as you get closer to your ideal weight." I didn't say "when you reach your ideal weight." This is very important. When you go on a diet you can't say you've succeeded until you reach your target weight. Most people who diet never reach their target weight, or if they do they quickly bounce back up again after they stop dieting.

Easyway is not a diet and does not involve setting a target weight. I've said you'll know you've achieved your ideal weight when you can admire what you see in the mirror and feel full of energy and happiness, but you don't have to wait for that moment before you can say you've succeeded and start enjoying life. The happiness kicks in as soon as you know you're no longer a slave to junk. You will quickly feel the cycle of misery change to a cycle of happiness as soon as you escape from the trap and start following Mother Nature's Guide.

THERE IS NOTHING TO WAIT FOR

SOWING SATISFACTION

When a gardener plants her bulbs ready for the following spring, she goes to bed happy that she's done what she needed to do to get the result she wants next year. She doesn't sit around feeling unfulfilled until all the flowers have come up and bloomed.

The knowledge that you've set in motion a process that will yield beautiful results is enough to trigger the cycle of happiness. It's when you know that you're neglecting your best interests but can do nothing about it that you feel miserable.

The change in mindset can happen overnight, but the physical changes that occur in the human body are very gradual by nature. Like watching the hour hand on a clock, we don't notice our hair growing longer or grayer, or our skin aging or our weight changing from one day to the next. If we did, we would not slide so passively into obesity; we would be shocked into doing something about it.

Your body was designed to change gradually and this is a vital aspect of Easyway. Its essential strength is that it's based on firm foundations. It will enable you to achieve dramatic improvements in fitness, health, and appearance, but it is not one of those methods that claims to do all that overnight. Anything that puts your body through such a rapid transformation will leave it in a state of shock and vulnerable to crash—like a castle built on sand. The gradual approach of Easyway makes it both painless and enjoyable; it also makes it permanent.

The pounds will start falling off from the moment you change your mindset and start following Mother Nature's Guide, but you won't necessarily notice the physical change from one day to the next. This is where your scale can come in handy. There's no harm in giving yourself further encouragement after you escape the junk trap and your scale can record the small changes that your brain can't detect from week to week.

A belt can also become your best friend as you start to lose weight. The happiness of gaining control over your eating is made even greater when you find that your clothes no longer fit—not because they're too tight but because they're too loose! Your belt starts to act as a tape measure. First you find you can tighten it by an extra hole, then another and another until you're having to make new holes in the belt! Each hole you cut will give you a tremendous high.

Incentives such as these are an essential part of Easyway, providing regular proof that the method works and that it is working for you.

> The same method (Easyway) is applicable to both men and women, but men and women are affected differently by the issue of food. For example, far more women than men have tried to diet and some have spent their lives constantly yo-yo dieting.
>
> Lots of double standards operate against women in society, including the pressures on them regarding food and overeating. Women who come to Easyway centers

often tell us the following:

- weight can become an obsession because of the stigma of being overweight
- when you feel overweight, a sense of shame begins to attach itself to eating
- a vicious circle follows: insecurities develop, bound up with the feeling of "not looking good," and women then seek comfort in overeating
- women become sensitive when remarks are made about their appearance, or perceive slights where none may have been intended
- women's views of themselves are often harsher than men's, including regarding body image (though this may be changing as men's bodies become more objectified), and they develop low self-esteem
- food becomes a constant temptation: Women tend to spend more time around food than men (as chief provider for the family) and it is available to them at all hours if they're at home
- diets are always negative for women. That's why there are no targets with Easyway: The key is to change the way you think and, from this, the right behavior will naturally follow
- women often come to regard food as a crutch when things go wrong: breaking up with a boyfriend, for example, means "Get out the cake and the ice cream,

> or buy a box of chocolates"—but this does not make them feel better
> - women often begin concealing the amount they have eaten from other members of the family—some start eating guiltily on their own in the kitchen
> - the feeling of unattractiveness caused by overeating can lead to depression and anxiety.

ONE-THIRD OF YOUR PROBLEM SOLVED

No doubt you're eager to press on and start experiencing this cycle of happiness for yourself. Rest assured, I'm not holding you back. You've already begun the process and should be feeling elated at what you stand to achieve.

Let's recap the instructions so far:
- FOLLOW ALL THE INSTRUCTIONS IN ORDER
- KEEP AN OPEN MIND
- START OFF WITH A FEELING OF ELATION
- DISREGARD ANY ADVICE THAT GOES AGAINST MOTHER NATURE'S GUIDE
- DISPENSE WITH ANY TARGET WEIGHT.

You have every reason to be feeling excited and elated because you already have one third of your problem solved. You've understood and accepted that it is counterproductive to set yourself a target weight.

You've thrown away that particular stick to beat yourself with and can get on with enjoying your life, content in the knowledge that, simply by starting the program, you've set yourself on the way to being the weight you want to be—the weight that you happen to be when you look at yourself in the mirror and admire what you see. Your bulbs are planted; there's no need to wait for the bloom.

So let's press on and examine the other two-thirds of the problem.

SUMMARY

- **A target weight serves no useful purpose. It can be a stick to beat yourself with or a convenient excuse for failure.**

- **Why set a target you don't believe in? Your eyes and lungs will tell you when you're the weight you want to be.**

- **Fourth instruction: DISPENSE WITH ANY TARGET WEIGHT.**

- **Easyway is gradual, painless, and enjoyable. It's also permanent.**

- **Use your scale, clothes, and belt to chart your progress.**

- **You've already solved one-third of your problem. The sense of achievement starts now.**

CHAPTER 7

FUELING UP AND BURNING OFF

IN THIS CHAPTER
- *WHY YOU PUT ON WEIGHT*
- *EXERCISING TO LOSE WEIGHT* • *WHY WE EAT*
- *TAKING CONTROL OF INTAKE*

Why do we treat our bodies differently from the way we treat our cars? Both need fuel for the same reasons.

OK, let's get down to basics. Why do you think you put on weight? No doubt it's a question you've asked yourself many times, usually out of exasperation, but we're not talking about the reasons you've found it impossible to control your weight in the past; we're talking about the simple physical equation that results in weight gain.

You don't need to be a physicist or biologist to know that a body will gain weight if you add more to it than you take away. In other words, you gain weight when your intake exceeds your disposal.

It's as simple as that.

Don't be distracted by any other reasons you might hear that try to explain why people weigh more than they want to:

glandular problems, a slow metabolism, a lack of exercise. These factors may well have some bearing on your weight, but they are not the fundamental cause of weight gain. The simple fact is that nothing grows without being fed.

It may well be the case that you have a physiological condition, be it glandular, metabolic, or something else, that means you can't eat as much as the next person, but this doesn't mean you must deprive yourself of the food you want when they don't have to. Going back to the car analogy, is it a problem if a friend's car consumes more fuel per mile than yours does? Of course not. Both cars consume the fuel they need to get from A to B. If you follow Mother Nature's Guide and ignore any conflicting advice, as instructed in Chapter Five, you'll be able to eat as much as you want, regardless of your glands or metabolic rate.

A lack of exercise is often cited as the main reason people become overweight. "If she didn't sit around all day..." Overweight people are generally regarded as lazy, while energetic people like sportswomen, dancers, and others who make a career out of vigorous exercise certainly give the impression that weight isn't a problem for them.

But don't be fooled. Exercise creates an increased need for food and if those people ate as much as they wanted to, they would be much bigger than they are. They deprive themselves of the food they crave because their livelihood depends on it.

EXERCISE IS NOT A GUARANTEED WAY TO LOSE WEIGHT

And neither is a lack of exercise the reason for putting on weight. If it was, wouldn't the snake be shaped more like a hippopotamus? Snakes lie around doing nothing most of the time, yet they remain long and thin and capable of incredible speed and agility when they need it. Big cats spend most of their time sleeping, but they don't become overweight and lose the ability to run and capture prey. They might go for a long time barely raising an eyebrow, yet they remain exactly the size and shape they were designed to be, simply by maintaining an equal balance between their intake and disposal.

HOPELESSNESS OF THE LONG-DISTANCE RUNNER

There's a common scenario among people who come to me for help with losing weight. I get men and women who've decided to take up running and have set themselves a target, such as a marathon or half-marathon, somewhere in the future. They feel enthusiastic about the effort involved because they believe it will help them shed a few pounds, as well as giving them a sense of achievement.

So they begin their disciplined routine of running every day and this can go on for months leading up to their target event. They do the run, feel great about their achievement, but when they get home and stand on the scales they find they haven't shed a single pound! Despite all those miles on the road, pounding the streets to get fit for the race, they've lost absolutely no weight at all.

It sounds incredible and yet they never seem unduly surprised. They admit that, deep down, they knew they hadn't lost any weight. They could feel it. For every ounce that they'd burned off pounding the roads, they'd eaten and drunk more than ever before to satisfy their increased hunger.

What drives a lion to wake up and hunt? Hunger. And when does it stop feeding? When its hunger is satisfied. You apply the same principles when putting fuel in your car. You don't drive your car to affect its weight. You probably don't even know what your car weighs. Why should you? It weighs what it was designed to weigh. You're probably aware that when you put fuel in, the weight increases and when you drive around and burn fuel off the weight comes down, but do you care? That's not why you put fuel in, is it?

You don't drive your car around to reduce its weight. That would be ridiculous. But it is exactly what we do to our bodies when we put ourselves through special exercise in order to lose weight.

Please don't take this as an instruction to avoid exercise. That's not what I'm saying at all. Exercise is a wonderful form of recreation and I thoroughly encourage it because it makes you feel good. But if you do it out of a desire to control your weight, you'll spoil the fun.

WHY DO WE EAT?

The scientific answer to this question is that we'd die of starvation if we didn't. But when you sit down to a meal, do you always think to yourself, "I must eat this food to prevent myself from starving to death"? Of course not. So let's now think about the feelings that compel us to eat.

If someone tapped you on the shoulder as you sat down to your evening meal and asked you why you were about to eat the food in front of you, you'd probably shrug and reply that it's what you always do at this time of day. Asked the same question when you were buying a snack in the middle of the afternoon, you might answer that that was habit and routine too, or perhaps you'd say it was an impulse triggered by the aroma of cooking, or because you regard the snack as a source of enjoyment.

In fact, the most common reasons given for eating are:

Part of the usual routine

Giving way to temptation

Out of boredom

Because of restlessness

To be sociable.

There's nothing wrong with eating according to a routine. It's practical and it generally fits in with the times of day when you're genuinely hungry. But if the routine is too rigid, it can cause a problem.

Imagine you fueled your car according to the same routine by which you eat, putting in the same amount at the same time every day. Perhaps you drive a regular number of miles every day, and so you know that the fuel you put in will keep your car running for the desired distance, but what if you don't use the car one day? Will you still go and put your usual amount in the tank?

Of course not! And yet this is how we fuel up our bodies, sticking rigidly to a format that we've been conditioned to follow and paying no regard to the fluctuations in our daily activities? Why the difference?

With the car we know full well that the manufacturer intended us to put fuel in for no other reason than to make it run. They also fitted a fuel gauge so we could see when the tank's getting low and fuel up before it runs out. The leading expert on how the human body works is Mother Nature and she designed us to take in fuel for exactly the same reason as you put fuel in your car: in order to keep us functioning.

She also fitted us with a fuel gauge—hunger—and she happened to make the fueling process very enjoyable to help us make sure we took in the right type of fuel.

What makes you buy the food you do? The Pan-European Survey of Consumer Attitudes to Food, Nutrition and Health found that the top five influences on food choice in all European member states are:
"Quality/freshness"—74%
"Price"—43%

"Taste"—38%

"Trying to eat healthily"—32%

"What my family wants to eat"—29%

Females, older subjects, and "more educated" subjects considered health aspects to be particularly important. Males more frequently selected "taste" and "habit" as main determinants of their food choice. "Price" seemed to be most important with unemployed and retired subjects.

EATING ON IMPULSE

The temptation to eat a snack between meals has nothing to do with the need for fuel and everything to do with brainwashing. It's like stopping and fueling at every gas station you pass, regardless of how much you've already got in the tank, purely because you like gas stations. The temptation comes from the illusion that these snacks taste great. Yet we gobble them up so fast we don't have a chance to taste them. All they're doing is fulfilling a mental desire, created by brainwashing.

The fact that we eat in response to boredom and restlessness is also the result of brainwashing and is a sure sign that we're confused about what food can do for us. The illusion of a crutch makes us reach for the cookies or a chocolate bar when we're waiting for the time to pass or we're struggling with a piece of work that's becoming a drag. But when we've finished the snack and return to our work, the problem's still there. The snack hasn't relieved it at all.

And why on Earth should it? It's illogical, but we've been conditioned to believe that eating will relieve boredom and stress. These feelings are usually caused by a genuine problem, be it a piece of work that's proving difficult or a coming event about which we're feeling insecure, for example. Whatever the problem, it's not hunger. Yet we reach for a snack in order to comfort ourselves.

Our brainwashed minds make the connection that a problem that has nothing to do with hunger could be alleviated by eating, because that's how snacks have been sold to us.

"Need to unwind? Have a bath and a chocolate bar."

"Watching a tense drama? Eat some potato chips or popcorn."

Eating a cookie doesn't alleviate boredom and nerves any more than drinking a cup of water. Have you ever thought to yourself, "I feel nervous, I'll have a drink of water and that will make things better?"

SOCIAL EATING

In most cultures, food is a social grace and that's a wonderful thing. Mother Nature intended us to enjoy eating, which is why she made our favorite foods taste so delicious. But feeling obliged to eat when you're not hungry goes against nature and is no pleasure at all.

We return to the example of Christmas dinner. Just because everyone else has a plate piled high with food, we feel we have to follow suit and we end up feeling bloated and lethargic. If someone goes to the trouble of cooking us a meal, we feel obliged to finish it all. Then they feel obliged to offer us seconds and we feel obliged to accept! This isn't eating for pleasure. It's suffering to fit in.

Stop eating out of routine, temptation, boredom, restlessness, or to be sociable and start eating for the reasons Mother Nature intended and you'll begin to see how easy it is to balance your intake with your disposal.

TAKE CARE OF YOUR INTAKE AND THE REST WILL TAKE CARE OF ITSELF

Intake and disposal are the two sides of the equation that determines whether you gain weight, but you only need to concern yourself with one side: intake. As I've explained, there's no need to regulate your rate of disposal through special exercise, other than for your own enjoyment. There are fat creatures that burn off a lot of energy and thin creatures that burn off very little. The regulating factor is their intake.

It's the distance we have to drive that ultimately determines how much fuel we need to put in the tank, not the other way around. And if we go a week without using the car, we know not to put in any gas.

This is exactly how wild animals eat. The squirrel knows to stop eating nuts and start storing them when it's eaten enough to keep itself functioning. Humans are designed to work in the same way too, yet we've become so confused about this that we keep pumping in the fuel even when the tank is already full. The tail is wagging the dog.

And just as your gas tank will spill over if you overfill it, your body can't cope with the excess. In the case of the car, the gas splashes out all over the forecourt, but imagine if it overflowed from the tank into the trunk. That's effectively what happens with your body. When you overeat, the junk sloshes out of your normal fuel stores and into your midriff, buttocks, waist, chest, arms, legs, neck, and face, and sits there in unsightly bulges.

As we continue to examine the reasons why we get our fueling all wrong, it will help to remember the comparison between your body and a car. The car is there to get you from A to B as the need arises. That could be five miles; it could be 500 miles. It doesn't matter. All you need to do is make sure that you provide enough fuel for the journey. You don't need to worry about the car's unladen weight, or how it disposes of the fuel it burns. Your job is to maintain the car in good working order with the correct type of fuel and oil.

From now on you're going to apply this principle to your body. This is Mother Nature's principle—the way you were designed to eat. One day you might work very hard and burn off a lot of fuel; the next you might take a day off, maybe spend the afternoon sitting in the yard doing nothing at all. All you have to do is apply the same flexible approach to eating as you do to fueling your car. That's what wild animals do and they don't worry about their weight, or how they dispose of the food once they've digested it.

All they're concerned about is finding a sufficient supply of their favorite food.

SUMMARY

- **You gain weight when intake exceeds disposal.**
- **Exercising to lose weight is like driving to burn off gasoline.**
- **You refuel your car when it needs it; apply the same principle to yourself.**
- **Weight and disposal will take care of themselves if intake is correct.**

WHAT'S ON THE MENU?

We can solve your weight problem by focusing on your intake.

You've been promised from the start that this method will make it easy and enjoyable for you to lose weight. Our first task was to simplify the problem by removing any distractions. We've established that you don't need to worry about a target weight or the rate at which your body burns calories. You have just one thing to concentrate on: intake.

GET THE INTAKE RIGHT, AND DISPOSAL AND WEIGHT WILL FALL INTO PLACE

You don't have to be a mechanic to know that you shouldn't put diesel in a petrol engine and vice versa. The two types of engine work in different ways and are designed specifically to run on a certain type of fuel. But you don't need to know this.

All you need to know is the type of fuel that is required for your car and, of course, which fuel comes out of which pump.

These days they've made it harder to put diesel in a petrol engine by making the nozzle too big, but you can still do it the other way around and anyone who ever has will know what a pain it is. Engines don't take kindly to the wrong type of fuel. In fact, as cars have become more sophisticated they've become more particular about the type of petrol they consume. If you want to keep your car running at peak performance, you just have to know which type of fuel it prefers and make sure that's the one you use. Get it wrong and your car will underperform. Get it badly wrong and it will break down.

The human body is a lot more resilient than any car engine. Put diesel in a petrol engine and it will stop working almost immediately, but if a child swallows a tiny plastic toy you're unlikely to notice any visible symptoms other than mild alarm! Some people make a living out of eating all sorts of rubbish—there was even a man who ate an entire airplane! That's how resilient the human digestive system is, but the danger is that this misleads us into thinking we can get away with eating anything we like. Treat your stomach like a waste disposal unit and it will suffer. It may not stop you in your tracks, as diesel will stop a petrol car, but it will slow you down.

When we stray from the foods that Mother Nature designed for us, we become heavy, slow, and lethargic. Heartburn, constipation, diarrhea, stiff joints, and tooth decay are among the more uncomfortable symptoms, and as your digestive system tries to cleanse itself, pushing anything it is not designed to burn into out-of-the-way places so that its vital organs can continue to function, the impurities gather as unsightly fat deposits and harmful chemicals, suffocating your muscles, damaging your skin, and clogging up your bloodstream. Over time, more life-threatening conditions develop: heart disease, high blood pressure, diabetes, cancer, obesity. Eventually, like an ill-used engine, it all grinds to a halt.

The aim of telling you all this is not to frighten you out of eating junk but to get rid of any belief that you can live on junk and get away with it. Don't wait for those life-threatening symptoms to develop: Your body is already suffering and you'll be amazed how much better you feel when you stop eating junk. It's like the difference between an old jalopy that splutters and backfires, and runs like a snail, and a brand new limousine that purrs smoothly at full power with no apparent effort at all.

GROWING OLD PAINFULLY

The so-called "baby boomer" generation is supposed to have been the most blessed in history. It is the generation that grew up in the wake of World War II, enjoying the benefits of a world of change, combining great advances in technology and medicine with greater opportunities for travel and socializing, a less hidebound approach to life, and a revolution in the supply and preparation of food.

You could say it was a generation that saw humankind

progress very quickly in a short space of time. Yet today there's clear evidence that the baby boomers are suffering more than previous generations due to health problems such as aching joints, asthma, diabetes, and strokes.

Why should this be? While the average lifespan is increasing because of the growing use of drugs to keep people alive, the actual health of our older population appears to be getting worse. Could it be that this generation also served as the guinea pigs for the explosion of processed food that has led to today's obesity and diabetes epidemics?

NATURE'S MENU

Wild animals avoid all these health problems by sticking to the fuel designed for them by Mother Nature. Every creature on the planet has developed its own specific diet and with it the physical attributes to handle that diet. (Note that the word "diet" in this instance has a very different meaning from the way it is used in relation to weight loss. An animal's diet consists of the correct amount of its favorite foods; a weight loss diet consists of the incorrect amount of all sorts of different foods.)

Mother Nature's plan is an incredibly complex system designed with one very important purpose:

SURVIVAL

Unlike modern humans, wild animals have always had to compete for food. If Mother Nature had designed every animal to eat the same diet, the biggest and strongest among them would thrive and the smallest and weakest would die. That in turn would cause the biggest and strongest to die because they depend on the smallest and weakest in many ways. For example, the largest creature on the planet, the blue whale, feeds on one of the smallest, plankton.

So Mother Nature has given every creature a chance to survive by presenting it with its own food packages that it can enjoy without too much competition. She has then developed us all with the physical attributes to access that diet. The legs and neck of the giraffe, the trunk of the elephant, the snout of the anteater, the teeth and claws of the lion—these are all physical features that have evolved to assist the animal in getting hold of its favorite food.

Just as all creatures have developed the tools with which to obtain their food, they've also developed the internal organs with which to digest it. The cow, for example, has a much more complex stomach than our own, consisting of four different sections. These developments have not happened overnight; they've evolved over millions of years to adapt to the food available. The giant panda was originally a carnivore and it still has vestiges of its carnivorous past, yet at some point in history it was presented with the need to find an alternative food and it developed the stomach for bamboo.

It's a fragile but ingenious ecosystem that is designed to bend and flex with natural conditions and evolutionary changes, apart from when people come along and stick a wrench in the works. We are the only creatures on the planet that don't adhere to Mother Nature's Guide. For some reason, we think we know better, even when our clumsy actions threaten our own existence and the existence of other creatures we love. The giant panda is in danger of becoming extinct because it has had its habitat destroyed and its food supplies stripped away. The disappearance of wildlife from land that has been savaged by humankind is not a flaw in Mother Nature's plan; it's the consequence of us thinking we know best.

OUR NATURAL DIET

The giant panda evolved from a meat eater into a plant eater, but it cannot evolve fast enough to cope with the restrictions imposed by humankind. And neither can we. The evidence of the baby boomer generation is that the mass consumption of processed foods is having a catastrophic effect on our health. Perhaps you think this is an exaggeration; we're hardly facing extinction! But this book is not talking about the base survival of the human race; it's talking about happiness and quality of life. Enjoying the way you eat is fundamental. There is plenty of evidence—and you've witnessed it first hand—that our diet of processed food is the cause of untold misery.

Animals don't have to undergo special exercise to maintain their ideal weight, nor do they have to know what their ideal weight is. All they have to take care of is their intake. Does it not follow that for you to free yourself from dietary problems and achieve your ideal weight, you need to follow the example of the rest of the animal kingdom?

Perhaps you're thinking, "So is this the point where you tell me I have to give up all my favorite foods and live off lettuce?"

Not at all. The aim of this book is to make eating enjoyable again and to help you lose weight easily and painlessly. It's not about making you sacrifice anything. It is about free choice. You can choose everything you eat—the only difference is that it will be an informed choice, not one made in a fog of brainwashing. Your choice will not be informed by Easyway but by Mother Nature's Guide—the leading authority on what is, and isn't, good for you to eat.

This is why the second instruction is so important. It's essential that you keep an open mind and don't allow your intellect to override your instincts.

Is your mind still open? Good!

So let's imagine you did follow the example of the animals and stopped eating processed foods. That means nothing that's been refined, frozen, pickled, preserved, smoked, sweetened, flavoured, mixed, added to, or cooked.

"Whoa! Wait a minute. You're telling me I can't cook!"

I'm not imposing any such restrictions. You can go on cooking, adding seasonings, and delicious sauces to your heart's content. All I'm asking now is that you put away your preconceptions and think about the foods that would be available to you if you followed Mother Nature's Guide, i.e. foods that require no cooking or processing yet taste wonderful without any need for flavorings, seasoning, or sauces. Do you agree that it comes down to fruit, vegetables, nuts, and seeds?

When you stop to think about it there is a vast array of foods available to us that requires no processing at all. But our tendency is to tamper with even the simplest of meals. When you come home at the end of the day, you might opt for a quick snack of jam on toast. It seems simple enough. But look closer at the human intervention involved in the making of that snack.

First the bread: a mixture of milled and refined flour, yeast, salt and numerous additives, baked in an oven. Next the butter: processed from cow's milk—natural enough for calves, maybe —then pasteurized, homogenized, churned, and refrigerated to prevent it from decomposing. The jam is made by boiling the life out of fruit mixed with a large quantity of refined sugar and preservatives. All that for a slice of toast and jam! Alternatively, you could just have a banana.

There are few things more enticing than the smell of hot toast, so you might argue that all this tampering is for the better. But does it really improve the foods in question? Or does it merely remove any nutritional value that the individual ingredients had to begin with? Cooking food has been shown to destroy important vitamins, most notably B and C, as well as breaking down proteins and destroying some antioxidants and essential fatty acids.

But I promised that you wouldn't be ordered to stop cooking your favorite meals, nor made to stick to a diet of fresh fruit, vegetables, nuts, and seeds. These foods just happen to be the ones designed for us by Mother Nature and they also happen to be the most tasty, but they're not the only foods we're capable of eating. Mother Nature is much more flexible than that.

It's time to introduce you to the "Junk Margin."

THE JUNK MARGIN

It's quite possible that when you finish this book, you'll decide that a diet of nothing but fresh fruit, vegetables, nuts, and seeds is to your liking, and what a healthy and energetic life you'll lead if that's the case. But the aim of Easyway is not to put you on any kind of diet at all; it's to show you the truth about the food you eat now so that you can make your own free choice, which in turn will lead to you enjoying life and the way you eat more than you do now. We can be quite flexible about this because Mother Nature's ingenious design hasn't restricted us exclusively to these unprocessed foods. There's a built-in margin for error, which enables us to eat a certain amount of "second-rate" foods without doing ourselves harm.

It's part of the survival plan that enabled the giant panda to evolve from a carnivore to a herbivore. When our favorite foods are scarce, Mother Nature enables us to get the nutrients we need from other sources. Thanks to this margin for error we're able to eat meat, fish, grains, and other processed foods, and derive some nutritional value from them. The margin for error is different for all species. The koala bear, for example, is limited exclusively to eucalyptus leaves (fortunately for them there are numerous different kinds of eucalyptus tree), whereas the goat can eat almost anything, meat or vegetation. But no other animal on the planet can match the variety of the human diet.

Not only are we able to eat meat, vegetables, fruit, and fish, we can also combine this mixture within the same meal, even in the same mouthful. The human digestive system has evolved to cope with this wide range of foods and cleverly sort it into nutrients and waste, but don't be misled into thinking it does so without a struggle. The Junk Margin was designed to be a fallback for when our favorite foods were not available. Through the intellectual exploitation of food-processing techniques, it has become our mainstay and we are suffering as a result.

Please don't misunderstand what the Junk Margin is. In this context it doesn't mean pizza or a Big Mac and fries, or a Krispy Kreme doughnut. The food that makes up your Junk Margin should be our secondary foods such as meat, fish, dairy etc. I'll explain more about what kind of food can be consumed as your Junk Margin later.

The Junk Margin is a wonderful asset in our survival and it will be a useful aid in helping you to take control of the way you eat, but it's very important to remember:

THE JUNK MARGIN IS EXACTLY THAT: A MARGIN

It is not designed to be, and should never become, the mainstay of your regular diet. Just because your stomach has developed the ability to process all the different things you throw at it, don't be fooled into thinking you can just put any old food in your mouth and expect your digestive system to cope. It's an abuse of the human body that we call "the plastic bucket syndrome."

SUMMARY

- It's important to understand the effects of incorrect eating.
- All animals were designed to eat specific foods for survival.
- The foods designed for us are fresh fruit, vegetables, nuts, and seeds. These are our favorites.
- The Junk Margin enables us to survive when our favorite foods are unavailable; it was not designed to be the mainstay of our regular diet.

Chapter 9

THE PLASTIC BUCKET SYNDROME

IN THIS CHAPTER

•ONE PART OF THE STORY
•HOW DO HERBIVORES GET THEIR PROTEIN?
•THE DIGESTIVE PROCESS •COUNTING THE CALORIES
•MISGUIDED CHOICES

The brainwashing confuses us into eating harmful foods because we think they're necessary for our health. We've only been given one side of the story.

Imagine your car ran out of gas miles from the nearest garage and a passer-by told you, "Don't worry, your car runs on gas, which is a by-product of crude oil. There's a plastic bucket in my trunk. Plastic also happens to be a by-product of crude oil. We can cut the bucket up and push the pieces into your gas tank. The engine will do the rest."

Would you thank them very much for their advice? Or would you flag down the first car you saw and tell them you were being pestered by a lunatic?

The suggestion that you might put a chopped-up plastic bucket into the fuel tank of your car is clearly ridiculous, yet we shove junk down our throats on much the same basis. For example, two of the minerals we need from our diet are calcium and iron. A piece of chalk contains calcium: would you eat a piece of chalk? Would you eat an iron nail? Unless you're a circus performer, it's safe to assume you wouldn't.

IN HER OWN WORDS: THERESA'S STORY

Up to the age of 45 I took a very cavalier approach to eating. I was always overweight, but I shrugged it off and told myself that I was just one of those people who preferred to live well and die young, rather than stay alive to a grand old age but not actually live at all. Who was I kidding? Did I really consider my constant feeling of tiredness to be "living well?" How can you live well when the slightest exertion leaves you out of breath? Worse than that, I regularly suffered from indigestion and constipation, which slowed me down even more.

That was my physical state; mentally I was even more of a mess. Just about every time I ate I felt guilty. I would indulge in these binges like a schoolgirl having a midnight feast and then I'd feel terrible as soon as it was over. If I tried to stop myself, I just felt deprived. This was my state of mind every single day!

Looking back, it seems incredible that I let myself get into that condition. I put all my effort into convincing myself that it was OK, rather than doing something to change it. That's because I honestly thought I had no choice. I believed it was just the way I was made, so it came as a revelation to learn that I did have a choice. It makes me quite angry, actually, to think that I was brainwashed for so long. I suffered unnecessarily for years and it was only when I discovered Easyway that I learned the truth.

I feel like someone who has escaped from an abusive relationship, the only difference being that the abuse was self-inflicted. I endured it for years because I thought it was the only life available to me. Now I know there's no need to suffer—we're not born to be unhappy—and I have a level of happiness in my life that I never realized existed. I used to think that healthy eaters couldn't be as jolly as they made out. I suspected it was a front. But it was me who was putting on the front. Now I'm free of all that nonsense and it feels wonderful to be alive.

Here's another example of the Plastic Bucket Syndrome. As any nutritionist will tell you, we need protein to build muscle. Meat is a rich source of protein. So we eat meat, convinced that if we didn't we would suffer a protein deficiency. Where do we get the meat from? Cows, sheep, pigs, chickens. Those are our main sources. Do you ever stop to wonder where those animals get their protein from? Cows aren't meat eaters, yet they're considerably bigger and stronger than we are—how on Earth do they do it?

While we're thinking big, what about elephants, rhinos,

giraffes, hippos, horses, buffalo, gorillas... Most of the largest and strongest animals on land are strictly plant eaters but they're clearly not suffering from a deficiency of protein. You have to ask yourself where we get the idea that we should eat meat for protein. Is it from Mother Nature's Guide? Or is it from scientists, who in turn get their information from other scientists?

By turning to meat for our protein, we're falling foul of the Plastic Bucket Syndrome. We haven't been given the full story. Obviously, it's possible to get protein, and plenty of it, from sources other than meat, but we're brought up believing meat is our best source of protein. Similarly, we're told to consume dairy products to get the calcium we need, but it's no more natural for humans to drink cow's milk and eat cheese than it is to eat a piece of chalk.

We need calcium to build strong bones and teeth. A bull elephant has strong bones and teeth. Ever seen a bull elephant eating cheese? It's laughable. The plain fact is that an elephant gets its immense tusks, its size, its energy, and its strength from eating only vegetation.

Think about it for a moment. There isn't a single species of animal that continues to consume milk beyond infancy. To do so is not only unnecessary, but is entirely unnatural. Yet nutritionists and scientists have maintained for decades that dairy food is an essential part of our adult diet. There's absolutely nothing scientific about that!

VEGAN ALERT!

At this point you may be starting to feel uneasy. "You're going to try and turn me vegan!" No, I'm not. Remember the Junk Margin? I'm not here to restrict you in any way. By explaining that you don't need meat for protein or milk or dairy produce for calcium, I'm merely giving you an illustration of the false logic in the advice we're all given by so-called experts such as doctors, scientists, and nutritionists.

WHAT THE EYES DON'T SEE

It's vital that you understand that, whatever your body needs, it's not OK to put an amount of it in your mouth and forget about it. Just because you can no longer see what's going on once you've swallowed it, that doesn't mean the process is complete.

Your digestive system is incredibly complex—far more complex than the system that turns gas into power in a car. It begins at the chewing stage, where saliva mixes with the food in the mouth and starts to break it down. Once the food reaches the stomach, the digestive juices break it down further. Unlike a car engine, the stomach has the ability to react to different foods, adjusting both the juices and the digestion time accordingly. When it's done its best, the food is passed into the intestines where the vital elements are extracted and distributed around the body, with the remainder passing out as waste.

The last part of the process, where the nutrients are distributed around the body, is the equivalent of the explosion that powers your car engine and it can only take place effectively if the food has been properly digested. Any food that isn't included in

Mother Nature's Guide makes digestion harder and thus affects the performance of your body's engine. It will run slowly, it will labor, it will burn fuel inefficiently, and it will demand more. Eventually, it will grind to a halt.

MORE THAN YOU CAN CHEW

Before the days of electronic communication, our ancestors passed knowledge from person to person and from generation to generation in the form of songs, poems, and sayings. It was a way of making the information memorable and it certainly worked—many of these sayings are familiar to us today. We hear them from our parents when we're young, then we forget about them as we go through our young adulthood, but when we have children of our own we suddenly find ourselves saying the exact things our parents said to us, reciting the same sayings word for word.

There's wisdom in these sayings and they were born out of experience. When it comes to our eating habits, there are many old sayings that are designed to help us cope with the strain we put our bodies through. "Don't bite off more than you can chew," is one example. Chewing is important if you want to avoid indigestion and constipation. You may have heard the adage, "Chew each mouthful 100 times," but different foods require quite different amounts of chewing. Have you ever tried chewing a mouthful of ripe plum, pear, or peach 100 times? There's really no need.

We only need to thoroughly chew foods that are difficult to digest. Often chewing isn't enough. First we have to remove any indigestible parts and then cook the food to give us a better chance of being able to break it down. Does this sound like a natural process to you?

WHAT'S ON THE LABEL?

You may have been persuaded to try and make your diet healthier by paying special attention to the vitamin content of everything you eat, or counting the calories, or trying to insure that your diet is well balanced. It's a tedious task that rather takes the joy out of eating. With Easyway, you can stop worrying about such details. Mother Nature's Guide has already taken care of all that. The Guide is designed to insure that you get all the calories, vitamins, and other nutrients you need in exactly the right balance. It's only because we've ignored Mother Nature's Guide for so long that these details have become an issue for us.

Our intelligence caused the problem and now we're trying to apply intelligence to solve it. But taking any sort of supplement, such as a vitamin pill, is also a case of the Plastic Bucket Syndrome. The quick and easy way to break the cycle is to go back to Mother Nature's original plan. It's hard to ignore the advice of highly trained, intelligent people like doctors and nutritionists, but remember that the ultimate authority on what's best for your body is the power that created it. Mother Nature provides all the vitamins and minerals we need in natural, unprocessed forms.

The fourth instruction was to disregard any advice that goes against Nature. So how can you tell if a piece of advice contradicts Mother Nature's Guide?

It's simple:

FOLLOW YOUR INSTINCTS

HEALTHY EATING HINTS FOR BUSY WOMEN

Think about what you're eating at the moment. What is your daily eating pattern? It's likely that you regularly eat badly at particular times of the day. Identifying those moments is key to remedying them.

Keep plenty of good healthy food in stock and have a plan for what you'll do when you need to eat on the run or for when your shopping plans fall apart because of work or family commitments. Not having a plan is what often leads to eating junk food.

Don't skip meals. Regular meals are a good basis for controlling what you eat. Missing meals can often lead to binge-eating junk food.

Don't leave bowls of candies around the house. Do not lead yourself into temptation by keeping chocolate in the fridge, or junk food in your cupboards. You don't need it in the house, so get rid of it.

When you're planning to eat out, choose what you're going to order before you go. Restaurant menus are designed to tempt you to eat junk. If you decide what you're planning to eat before you go, you don't even need to look at the menu.

Don't reach for food when you are fed up or depressed. It never helps the situation.

Just as common sense tells you it's ridiculous to put a chopped-up plastic bucket in the fuel tank of your car, as long as you keep an open mind it will also sound the alarm whenever you're given advice that goes against Nature. The trick is making sure you heed it.

The purpose of this chapter is not to give you a lesson in biology. After all, wild animals get by perfectly well without having to think about how their digestive system works. The point is that you don't need to think about it either, any more than you need to contemplate carburettors and valves to know how to keep your car running. The manufacturer has provided you with the necessary information. Wild animals don't need to know how their digestive system works because they follow Mother Nature's Guide.

The more we think about what we eat, the more susceptible we are to brainwashing. Where do we get our information from? Can we trust our sources? And what gives them the authority to tell us how best to look after our bodies? You might have complete faith in someone who has studied the human body, but do you really think they know better than Mother Nature, who actually designed the human body herself?

When you're told that meat is a rich source of protein and dairy a rich source of calcium, you're only being given one side of the story. The picture is not complete. What you're not being told about are the harmful effects of eating meat and dairy. You're lucky that the human body is so resilient. It can withstand the Plastic Bucket Syndrome for years without missing a heartbeat, but don't be duped into thinking it's coming through all that abuse unscathed.

BLUNTING YOUR EDGE

There are two types of people in this world: those who enjoy mowing the grass and those who hate it. You rarely find anyone in between. Some people find it an arduous task, while others find it wonderfully rewarding. The difference is almost undoubtedly down to the condition of their mower.

If your mower is blunt, you end up doing twice the amount of work for half the result. But a well-adjusted, sharpened mower will breeze through the job with ease and leave a beautiful finish. If this sounds like an analogy for the human body when put to work, that's quite deliberate. When we're fit and sharp, physical challenges become a source of pleasure. When we're out of shape, even the simplest task becomes a chore.

If you've ever run your nice sharp mower over a stone, you'll know how painful that sound is. It's the sound of damage being done. That stone will have blunted the nice sharp edge of part of the blade and every time that happens the mower will become less efficient. Unlike the mower, your body has the ability to repair itself, and so one small bit of damage will soon be remedied and everything will continue to work perfectly.

But imagine running your lawnmower over Brighton beach which consists entirely of large pebbles: How long do you think those blades would last? A diet of junk food is not like one stone hitting your blades; it's a relentless barrage of pebbles inflicting one piece of damage after another. Your body doesn't have time to regain its edge and your incredible machine becomes blunt, inefficient, and slow.

MISGUIDED CHOICES

One of the great mysteries of human behavior is that we spend so much time and money taking care of our cars, yet we subject our bodies to such abuse on a daily basis. We look after our hair, our skin, and take pride in the clothes we wear. But your body is far more precious than a car and what you feed it is far more important than what you look like. If you destroy your car, you can get another one. But we only get one body. So why do you think we treat it so badly? We're not stupid—our intelligence is what sets us above every other animal on the planet. The only explanation has to be that we don't realize we're doing it. Why? Because we rely for our information on sources that never give us the whole story.

The human body can recover from the occasional stone in the blades. That's why we're able to allow ourselves a Junk Margin and still keep in shape. It's the relentless barrage of junk that does the lasting damage. In order to stop that barrage you need to let go of your preconceptions about the food you eat.

FIFTH INSTRUCTION: IGNORE ANY ADVICE THAT CONFLICTS WITH MOTHER NATURE'S GUIDE

We're conditioned to take a very black-and-white view of what is and isn't good for us. On the one hand we see food; on the other we see poison. If it's not a known poison, we regard it as food and, therefore, all right to eat. But if you can see that not all products of crude oil are suitable for the tank of your car, you can also understand that not all foods are suitable for your body.

SUMMARY

- Just because a food contains nutrients that you need doesn't mean that the food is good for you.

- The strongest animals on Earth don't get their protein from meat.

- No animal on earth consumes milk beyond infancy—dairy products never exist in other animals' diet.

- To get the nutrients we need from food, it must be properly digested.

- Fifth instruction: IGNORE ANY ADVICE THAT CONFLICTS WITH MOTHER NATURE'S GUIDE.

- There's no need to think about how your body works if you follow Mother Nature's Guide.

- You do have a choice over what you eat.

Chapter 10

FIRST STEPS TO FREEDOM

The brainwashing creates a perception of junk food that makes escape seem impossible. Unravel the brainwashing and the way out becomes clear.

You've reached the halfway stage of this book, and if you've followed all the instructions so far you'll be feeling excited about getting to the end and enjoying the moment of revelation when you realize you're no longer a slave to junk eating. In the second half, I'll take you through the simple steps that will lead you to this moment, applying what you've learned to the way you eat. First, though, let's recap the key points that we've covered so far.

THE TRAP

You've been caught in a trap that has made it impossible for you to take control of your eating and get your weight down to where you'd like it to be. Each failed attempt to free yourself from the trap reinforces your belief that it's incredibly hard, if not impossible, to escape from.

Addiction is 1 percent physical and 99 percent mental, and it makes you believe relief can only come from the very thing that's keeping you trapped. The misery people feel when they can't conquer their weight problem is the helplessness of being trapped and feeling too weak to do anything about it.

THE WRONG METHOD

The only reason people find it hard to escape the trap is that they follow the wrong method. Any method that requires willpower, such as dieting or undergoing a course of special exercise, is doomed to failure because it doesn't tackle the real cause of the problem: the belief that you get some sort of pleasure or crutch from bad eating. In fact, the willpower method reinforces the belief that quitting is hard and that the inability to quit is a weakness in the person, not the method.

IT DOESN'T HAVE TO BE HARD

If you attempt to lose weight believing that it's going to be hard, it will be hard. It's the belief that quitting is not easy that makes it hard. Wild animals find it the most natural thing in the world to eat as much of their favorite food as they want, whenever they want, and maintain their ideal weight without having to diet or undergo special exercise. So will you if you follow Easyway.

> *"One cannot think well, love well, sleep well, if one has not dined well."*
> **Virginia Woolf, author**

THREE-PART PROBLEM

When you want to lose weight you will have three factors in mind: your target weight, your intake of fuel, and how you burn it off. You can forget about the first and the last. There is no need to set yourself a target weight; you'll know when you've reached your ideal weight by looking in the mirror and being happy with what you see and how you feel. Undergoing special exercise to burn off calories is as pointless as driving your car to burn off fuel. Added to which, the more you burn, the more you'll need to consume.

The factor that you need to focus on is intake. Get your intake right and the other two will fall into place.

YOU'VE BEEN BRAINWASHED

The fact that the most intelligent species on the planet happens to be the only one to suffer eating problems can only be explained by the fact that our intelligence has led us astray. There are plenty of examples of human intelligence leading to self-destruction: the way we eat is just one more.

We prefer to take the advice of fellow humans, rather than follow the example of animals that have no weight problems and heed the guidance of our creator. Whatever you believe that to be, it wasn't a doctor or a nutritionist.

The advice of so-called experts and the people who brought us up, mixed with the advertising of the food industry, creates a barrage of brainwashing that gives us a one-sided picture of the food available to us. The only way to really know what's good for you is to clear your mind of the brainwashing and go back to Mother Nature's Guide.

THE INSTRUCTIONS
- FOLLOW ALL THE INSTRUCTIONS IN ORDER
- KEEP AN OPEN MIND
- START OFF WITH A FEELING OF ELATION
- DISPENSE WITH ANY TARGET WEIGHT
- DISREGARD ANY ADVICE THAT CONFLICTS WITH MOTHER NATURE'S GUIDE

LET GO OF THE PAST

Until you reconnect with Mother Nature's Guide, you may find it hard to believe that something as simple as instinct can free you from your weight problem. You've been brainwashed into believing it's a complex problem that requires a lot of effort and willpower to overcome. The news that escape is actually very easy is not always immediately welcome, especially if you've spent years trying and failing the hard way.

Remember that prison I talked about in Chapter Two, the one with the heavy door? Imagine you'd spent years in that prison, convinced that the door was too heavy for you to open, and then one day someone showed you that the door could be opened with a minimum of effort. You'd have mixed feelings: On the one hand, you'd be delighted that you were finally getting out; on the other, you'd be grieving for all those wasted years.

This negative feeling is often enough to prevent us from taking the opportunity to escape. When we think of all the time we've spent suffering unnecessarily, it makes us feel foolish. No one likes feeling like a fool so we try to justify our mistake. We look for proof that we stayed in the prison for some good reason and the only justification we can find is the belief that the junk we were eating really did give us pleasure or a crutch. We refuse to believe what we can see with our own eyes and actually choose to stay in the trap.

It's essential that you don't make this mistake. Forget about the past and think about the life that awaits you in the future: a life of genuine happiness, where you enjoy meals without physical discomfort or guilt or shame, where you feel great about the way you look and feel. The prison door is swinging open, and so far you haven't had to make any special effort or apply any willpower. Just walk toward it and have no doubt about what you can see with your own eyes.

SIXTH INSTRUCTION: NEVER DOUBT YOUR DECISION TO QUIT

Trying to find a logical reason why you keep eating junk will only lead you deeper into misery. The trap gives you a twisted view of the logic, so it will never make sense. The first step to freedom from the prison is recognizing that overeating is not just a habit that you can't seem to kick; it's an addictive trap that you've been caught up in due to brainwashing.

This changes your whole way of looking at the problem. For the first time, you can see that it's not a weakness in your character that has kept you hooked; nor is it some magical quality in the junk you've been eating. When you can see these two crucial facts, the feeling of powerlessness and despair goes and you begin to see the easy way out.

"By eating many fruits and vegetables in place of fast food and junk food, people could avoid obesity."
David H. Murdock, philanthropist

HOW EASYWAY WORKS

The thing about Easyway that makes people skeptical is its utter simplicity. How can a problem as apparently complex as overeating have such a simple solution? You should now be able to see that the problem is not complicated at all; it boils down to incorrect eating and nothing more. The complexity lies in the tangle of brainwashing that prevents you from seeing the clear picture.

Easyway works by using plain logic to unravel the brainwashing and replace it with clear, rational understanding of the problem. The method is easy and painless, but above all it is permanent. There's no point in releasing yourself from a trap if you're only going to walk back into it again. We want you to be free forever. To do that we need to change your mindset.

People who are overweight are notorious for dieting and then piling the weight back on again. They're just like smokers and drinkers who are not fortunate enough to find Easyway, and who are therefore forever stopping and starting again. Quitting temporarily isn't quitting at all. You're still hooked, you're still a slave, and you're still unhappy. In fact, during those periods when you feel like you're controlling your eating, you're actually less happy than when you're overeating because you still crave the junk, but you can't have it.

Stopping and starting can become a joke. It's a way of covering up your embarrassment when you know that overeating has become an everyday fact of life. Brainwashed into believing that your slavery to eating is quite normal, you kid yourself that it's a reason why people like you. Too bad it makes you feel miserable.

From an early age, we're brainwashed into believing that junk food gives us some sort of pleasure or crutch. This is the part of your mindset that we have to change. You need to see that

EATING JUNK DOES ABSOLUTELY NOTHING FOR YOU WHATSOEVER

You may not be convinced of this yet, but you should at least be prepared to be convinced. If you're not, you haven't followed the second instruction.

Everybody, unless they've been brought up on a remote island with no contact to modern society, is subjected to the brainwashing, but not everybody becomes an overeater. So what's the difference between them and you? The obvious answer is that you overeat and they don't, but that doesn't complete the picture. We need to know why the brainwashing works on some people and not on others.

You may have asked the question yourself from time to time. How can anyone show such a lack of interest in foods that you can't resist? Why don't they feel the same desire as you?

You've just hit upon the fundamental difference between people who can't help tucking in and those who are perfectly happy not to: nonovereaters don't have the desire to eat junk. They don't have the desire because they're not hooked. They've avoided the vicious circle.

ADDICTION CREATES THE DESIRE

Before you become hooked you are subject to the brainwashing, but there is no addiction compelling you to fall for it. Whether you do fall for it or not comes down to a chance decision that will be influenced by a combination of factors. Everyone is exposed to different influences throughout their lives and the lucky few are influenced to resist that initial temptation. But they are the few. The vast majority of people fall for the brainwashing and spend their lives eating junk.

It's also true that people who don't fall for the brainwashing when they're young may well fall for it later in life. Just because they haven't fallen into the trap, doesn't mean they've seen through the illusion. All it takes is a change in circumstances and they can succumb.

It's once you've fallen into the trap that the desire kicks in. I've explained about the illusion of pleasure. It's actually the relief of the craving, which people who aren't hooked don't suffer. Therefore, they never experience the illusion of pleasure, and so they don't develop the desire.

To unravel the problem and remove the desire, you have to remove the craving. The only way to remove the craving is to stop eating the junk.

Once you've achieved this state of mind, you will actually be less vulnerable to falling for the brainwashing in future than someone who has never had an overeating problem. For them, the misinformation that junk food gives some sort of pleasure or crutch is still there in their mind; they just haven't chosen to find out because they've been quite happy living without it. But their situation could change. A trauma of some kind could see them turning to food for comfort at any point in their life, believing it will give them the pleasure or support they need. When you escape the trap with Easyway, that belief no longer exists.

EASYWAY DOES NOT REQUIRE THE POWER OF REASON TO OUTWEIGH TEMPTATION; IT REMOVES TEMPTATION ALTOGETHER

Stoppers and starters never remove the desire for junk, so they feel deprived while they're denying themselves their little pleasures. They fight this feeling of deprivation by applying all their willpower, but eventually their willpower gives out. The trap makes you miserable whatever you do: miserable when you're eating, miserable when you aren't.

Take away the desire for junk and you remove the sense of sacrifice. If you think that will be hard, it's because you have a distorted view of food. We're not born with the desire to eat junk; it's something we acquire through conditioning. We acquire it without noticing and we can remove it just as easily.

> *"I've found when all I'm eating is really fresh, healthy foods, I stop craving pizza and burgers."*
> **Lauren Conrad, fashion designer and author**

A CLEARER VIEW

By the time you finish this book, your frame of mind will be such that, whenever you think about eating junk, instead of feeling deprived because you can't have it, you'll feel overjoyed because you no longer have to eat it. You'll see junk food addiction for what it really is.

It's easy for us to recognize the heroin trap and what it stands for: ADDICTION! SLAVERY! POVERTY! MISERY! DEGRADATION! DEATH! Food is rarely portrayed in this light. We're not shown the victims whose lives are cut short by diabetes, obesity, cancer, or any of the other ailments caused by overeating; we're shown happy, beautiful, smiling people having fun or acting cool, showing no signs of strain or anxiety, enjoying all the pleasures that life has to offer. The message is straightforward: "Junk food makes you happy."

Hammer out a message enough times and it begins to stick, but you know the truth, which is why you're reading this book. You've seen for yourself the harm that incorrect eating causes. It's time to blow away the illusions once and for all, stop seeing bad eating as a pleasure or crutch, and focus on the true picture.

If you can look at a heroin addict and see the mistake she's making when she thinks the next fix will make everything all right, you're already on the way to solving your own problem. The aim of this book is to help you find the happiness that comes with being free from the slavery of overeating. I'll help you to see that eating junk does not relieve your misery at all; it's the cause of it. The trap is not a prison from which you can never escape— escape is easy, provided you follow the right method.

In deciding to read this book, you were telling yourself that you've had enough of the way you eat and the food that controls you. Perhaps you reached that point a long time ago but didn't receive the correct instructions to help you out. Like all overeaters, you want to stop falling for temptation and start living again without feeling like a slave. You also don't want to spend the rest of your life feeling deprived.

As you work your way through the second half of the book, you can look forward to achieving all that. However, there may still be obstacles standing in the way of you feeling completely confident about your chances of success. You may be experiencing a sense of entering the unknown and that can be a daunting sensation. We need to examine any lingering fears you may be feeling.

SUMMARY

- **Your problem is not a weakness in you, nor something magical in the food you crave. It's a trap.**

- **The first step to freedom comes from recognizing the trap you're in.**

- **In order to escape permanently, you must remove the desire to eat junk.**

- **See all food in its true light and you'll begin to remove the desire for junk.**

- **Sixth instruction: NEVER DOUBT YOUR DECISION TO QUIT.**

Chapter 11

FEAR

IN THIS CHAPTER
•*THE TUG-OF-WAR* •*FEAR OF FAILURE*
•*FEAR OF SUCCESS* •*ALL YOU HAVE TO GAIN*
•*REMOVE ALL DOUBTS*

Fear is a very powerful motivator, but when it pulls you in conflicting directions, the result is confusion and the inability to act.

At some point during your descent into the junk-eating trap, there comes a time when you begin to fear the physical damage that you're doing to yourself. You realize that you've lost control of your eating and you recognize that you need to stop. This is a powerful fear and it's often the trigger for an attempt to do something about it, but it seldom leads to success because it's counterbalanced by another fear: the fear of life without your little crutch.

If you believe all the myths about junk food—that it tastes great, that it's the cheaper option, that it comforts you, and makes you happy—it follows that you believe life will be empty and hard without it. So all junk-eaters find themselves in a tug-of-war of fear: afraid to go on eating as they do and afraid to quit.

In order to help you free yourself easily, painlessly, and

permanently, we have to remove all your fears concerning eating.

Fear should not be regarded as an enemy. It's a natural instinct, designed to protect us from real dangers by triggering the release of hormones that make us faster, fiercer, and stronger. But through our intellect we are also susceptible to fearing dangers that don't exist. What do we say if we see someone looking anxious? "Don't worry; it might never happen." We're susceptible to the fear of imaginary dangers and we can get so wrapped up in those fears that we stop seeing things as they really are.

The ability to imagine harmful scenarios is one of the great advantages of human intellect. We call it foresight. It's the power to recognize the potential for danger and thus safeguard against it. But what if your projected fears are based on false information? Say, one day you read that fruit causes cancer, you'd probably stop eating fruit. You'd also worry about the harm it's already done to you over the years. As a result of false information, you'd not only deprive yourself of something vital for your wellbeing, you would also make yourself unnecessarily anxious.

As consumers, we're bombarded with so many mixed messages about what is and isn't good for us, it's hard to know which fears to take seriously and which to disregard. The upshot is that we become inert, stuck between conflicting fears.

> *"I think it's very expensive not to eat healthy. Eating healthy is the only affordable option we have left."*
> **Marcus Samuelsson, chef**

According to the National Eating Disorders Association, the average American woman is 5 feet 4 inches tall and weighs 140 pounds. The average American model is 5 feet 11 inches tall and weighs 117 pounds. The model has become the ideal for all women to aspire to, and this causes many to feel inadequate about their appearance. Eating disorders such as anorexia nervosa, bulimia nervosa, and binge eating most often appear during adolescence or early adulthood, and females are more likely to develop them than males. Eating disorders aren't just about food. Food is used to feel in control of other feelings that may seem overwhelming. Feelings of low self-esteem tend to accompany eating disorders, along with depression and anxiety.

Social pressures on women to be thin push women to the limit. Once you understand this, and realize that it is much better for you to be you than to try and be somebody else, you will regain control of your life again and learn to eat healthy foods which will make you the weight you should be—the right weight for you.

FEAR OF FAILURE

Anyone who has tried and failed to do something about their weight problem will know that it leaves you feeling more firmly trapped than you did before. You've seen movies where prisoners are thrown into a cell and the door locked behind them. The first thing they do is run to the door and tug at the handle. This confirms their predicament: They really are locked in. Trying and failing to get your weight down has the same effect on the overeater. It reinforces the belief that you're trapped in a prison from which there is no escape.

This is a crushing blow. The addict who tells herself she'll get free one day, just not yet, always allows herself to believe that she will be able to do so when the time is right. The addict who tries and fails repeatedly can't kid herself any more. Many people conclude that the best way to avoid this misery is not to try to escape in the first place. As long as they never try that prison door handle, they'll always preserve the belief that it might just open when they want it to.

This is the twisted logic of addiction—all trying to escape will do is confirm that escape is impossible. You can see what a self-defeating argument it is, yet there are millions of intelligent people who continue to delude themselves into believing it's the best strategy. They prefer to continue suffering the misery of being overweight than risk the misery of failure. What they don't realize is the door only remains shut if you use the wrong method to open it.

What is it you're afraid of? Remaining in the overweight trap? So the fear of failure is the fear of remaining overweight. But you're already overweight, so you're fearing something that has already happened. If you continue to avoid even trying to escape, you guarantee that you will feel a failure for the rest of your life.

It's like an aspiring actress who never goes to auditions because she's afraid of being rejected. What would be her chances of landing a role as an actress? Zero.

BY PROTECTING YOURSELF FROM THE FEAR OF FAILURE, YOU GUARANTEE THAT YOU FAIL

For the actress who does attend the audition, fear of failure is a positive force. It focuses her mind, drives her to learn her lines and practise harder, and gives her an energy that's compelling to watch. The same is true for all of us: When channelled positively, the fear of failure can magnify our abilities.

By trying to change the way you eat, you give yourself a chance of success. By trying to change it with Easyway, you give yourself the best possible chance. By following all the instructions in order, from beginning to end, you cannot fail.

> *"In our fast-forward culture, we have lost the art of eating well. Food is often little more than fuel to pour down the hatch while doing other stuff – surfing the web, driving, walking down the street. Dining al desko is now the norm in many workplaces. All of this speed takes a toll. Obesity, eating disorders, and poor nutrition are rife."*
> **Carl Honore, author of** *In Praise of Slow*

FEAR OF SUCCESS

The fear of failure can prevent an attempt to change the way you eat, but the bigger problem is the fear of success. You might wonder how or why anybody would fear success. After all, isn't that what everyone craves?

It all depends what success represents in your mind. Long-term prisoners often reoffend soon after they've been released. You might assume this is because they're habitual criminals and haven't seen the error of their ways. To most of us it seems crazy to go and get yourself back in prison when you've just been given your freedom after so many years, but for many long-term inmates prison is the only life they know. The prospect of having to make their way alone on the outside is so daunting that they deliberately reoffend just to get themselves back inside as soon as possible.

They yearn for the "security" of the prison. Life on the outside is alien and frightening for them: It doesn't run to the same routine or the same guidelines; it's not what they know and they don't feel equipped to handle it.

When you're hooked on junk food, the prospect of life without your little crutch is also frightening. You've been convinced that it comforts you and makes you happy, that it's delicious, and a treat. You also believe that you'll have to go through some terrible trauma to get free of it and that, without it, you'll never have that feeling of happiness and reward that you think you get now.

You're tricked into believing that controlling what you eat is boring. Though you're well aware of the misery that overeating causes, you may have come to regard it as part of your identity. The jovial glutton. The cuddly friend. Forget it! Your friends love you that way because it makes them feel slim by comparison.

The fear of success is based on all the illusions that we've already dealt with. If you're afraid that life without all the junk will be dull and difficult, then you haven't yet seen through the illusions and you still believe it gives you pleasure or a crutch. If you've followed all the instructions and understood everything you've read so far, you'll know that eating junk does absolutely nothing for you and you won't be "giving up" anything when you stop. In fact, the opposite is true: You'll make many wonderful gains, one of which is no longer having to live in limbo between two fears.

WIN THE TUG-OF-WAR

With every addiction, fear is the tether that keeps you trapped and it tugs at you whichever way you turn. When you're not eating junk, you suffer the empty, insecure feeling that makes you panic and think life without junk will be unbearable. When you're eating junk, it makes you feel bloated, fat, and undesirable and you wish you weren't, plus you have to deal with the fear of the control that it has over you.

The fear of remaining a slave to junk food for the rest of your life, however long or short that may be, should be enough to make you do something about it, but the fear of failure and the fear of success keep you in the trap. It can appear to be a hopeless situation, but, in fact, it's very easy to escape because all these fears are caused by the same thing: junk food.

The solution is obvious:

TAKE AWAY THE JUNK AND THE FEAR GOES TOO

What will happen to your fears if you no longer have a desire to eat junk?

- Your fear of the harmful consequences of eating junk will stop because you're no longer eating it.
- The illusion of pleasure will disappear and you'll stop fearing life without it. In other words, the fear of success will stop.
- You'll realize that stopping is easy and your fear of failure will end.
- Your health will improve, you'll feel full of life, and you'll find it much easier to relax.

You may be thinking, "Wait. So you're telling me the answer to my weight problem is to stop eating junk? I could have told you that!"

That is exactly what I'm saying and, I agree, it is blindingly obvious, but why do so many people fail to see it? If you stop because you feel you should, you're responding to a fear and it won't work because you'll still believe that you're making a sacrifice. If you stop because you have no desire to continue, then you're not having to respond to anything. That's the easiest thing in the world.

You probably have no desire to pour ice-cold water down your back, but it doesn't require any effort to make sure you don't. It probably doesn't even cross your mind. When you have no desire to do something, it's easy to avoid it.

The aim of this book is to help you lose weight and to do that you need to stop eating junk. But unlike other methods, Easyway doesn't stop there. We want you to stop eating junk for the simple reason that you have absolutely no desire to eat junk. To achieve that state of mind we need to help you to see that

THERE IS NOTHING TO FEAR

> *"There's a great metaphor that one of my doctors uses: If a fish is swimming in a dirty tank and it gets sick, do you take it to the vet and amputate a fin? No, you clean the water. So I cleaned up my system. By eating organic raw greens, nuts, and healthy fats, I am flooding my body with enzymes, vitamins, and oxygen."*
> **Kris Carr, author**

That's the purpose of this chapter: To make you see through the fears that keep you in the trap and to help you understand that, when you take the junk out of your life, your fears will disappear too. Junk food is not a pleasure or crutch that you need to learn to live without for the good of your health; it's your worst enemy and it gives you absolutely nothing at all. You instinctively know this because it's been making you miserable, so open your mind and follow your instincts.

If you could get an impression of how you'll feel after you've escaped from the trap, you might wonder, "Will I really feel this good?" Your fear will be gone and you'll feel an incredible energy and glow. This is how we're designed by Nature to feel. The misery and lethargy are unhealthy states caused by bad eating.

If you don't recognize this feeling of elation from your previous attempts to get free, it's because you were having to use willpower. Somewhere in your mind you still believed you were making a sacrifice, so you never experienced the joy of being truly free. We've said repeatedly that the willpower method doesn't work. It's time to explain in more detail exactly why that is.

SUMMARY

- Junk eaters are pulled in two directions by a tug-of-war of fear.
- Succumb to the fear of failure and you guarantee failure.
- The fear of success is based on illusions.
- Remove the junk and you remove the fear.
- Open your mind to everything you stand to gain. There is nothing to fear.

CHAPTER 12

WILLPOWER

IN THIS CHAPTER

- *SEEING THINGS A DIFFERENT WAY*
- *ARE YOU ALWAYS WEAK-WILLED?*
- *HABIT OR ADDICTION* •*OTHER DIETERS*

The widespread belief that you can't lose weight without using willpower is one of the major reasons why people find it so hard.

Most women who want to lose weight believe that it will be hard. They also believe that they'll stand no chance of succeeding unless they're strong-willed about it, so they make an attempt to do so by applying all their willpower and find it's incredibly hard. They draw the conclusion that they lack the necessary willpower to lose weight.

But look at the situation another way. If those women who find it hard to lose weight are using willpower, doesn't that suggest that it might be the use of willpower that makes it hard?

The trouble is that most women who try and fail to lose weight with the willpower method don't look at it this way. Why would they? Every organization with an interest in the way we eat, from governments and medical institutions to diet brands and the food industry, tells them that changing their diet requires willpower.

People who try to change the way they eat with the willpower method never win the tug-of-war of fear. On one side, their rational mind knows they should stop eating junk because it's making them overweight, sapping their energy, making them ill, controlling their life, and causing misery. On the other side, their addicted brain makes them panic at the thought of being deprived of their little crutch. It's this conflict that makes it hard to quit. Whether you eat junk or not, you're guaranteed to remain miserable. When you're not eating junk, you feel deprived, and when you do eat junk, you wish you didn't have to.

The willpower method requires you to focus on all the reasons for stopping and hope you can sustain your efforts long enough for the desire to go eventually. But as long as you continue to believe that junk food gives you pleasure or a crutch, the desire will never go.

The key is to remove the desire to eat junk. Do that and quitting is as easy as pushing open a door. But if you've ever come across a door with no handle and pushed on the wrong side, where the hinges are, you'll know how even the simplest of tasks can be hard if you go about it in the wrong way. The door might budge a tiny bit, but it won't swing open. It requires a huge amount of effort and determination. Push on the correct side and the door opens without you even having to think about it.

ENCOURAGING SOMEONE TO LOSE WEIGHT THROUGH THE USE OF WILLPOWER IS LIKE TELLING THEM TO OPEN A DOOR BY PUSHING ON THE HINGES

The need for willpower implies a conflict of will. You wish you could stop eating junk, but you don't want to live without eating junk. It's a conflict you cannot resolve through sheer willpower; it can only be resolved by removing one half of the tug-of-war: the desire to keep eating junk.

ARE YOU ALWAYS WEAK-WILLED?

So you try and fail to quit with the willpower method and, rather than blame the method, you blame yourself for not having the strength of will. For many women, this is very upsetting because they pride themselves on their strength of will in other situations. They can bring up children, run companies, lead a country—sometimes all three!—yet here they are feebly overpowered by the temptation to eat a cake!

How can you be strong-willed in one aspect of your life and weak-willed in another? Is willpower really selective?

Women who eat a diet of junk have often shown a strong will to get to that stage, especially if that diet includes oysters, blue cheese, coffee, or alcohol, for example. It takes a strong will to be able to consume all these things without wanting to be sick. Remember I talked about acquiring a lack of taste? That takes perseverance and determination.

Many of the foods and drinks that we come to regard as favorites take some getting used to at first. It's the body's natural defenses doing their best to reject harmful substances. But because we've been brainwashed into thinking these foods are pleasurable, we push ourselves to like them. The willpower required to overcome the natural aversion to poisons like caffeine, alcohol, and nicotine is huge.

Furthermore, isn't it your will to keep junk in your life that's driven you to carry on eating it despite the powerful arguments to quit eating it, and indeed your own desire to do so? When you stop and think about it, there's plenty of evidence to show that overeaters are actually very strong-willed, not weak-willed.

The same is true of smoker and drinkers—the same applies with all addictions: It takes a strong will to overcome the revulsion and get hooked, and it takes a strong will to stay hooked in the face of all the reasons to stop. Of course some people end up being smokers, drinkers, and junk eaters.

There is a connection between multiple addictions, but it's not that they're signs of a lack of willpower. On the contrary, they're more likely evidence of a strong will. What they all share is that they're traps created by brainwashing. And one of the biggest pieces of brainwashing is that quitting requires willpower.

ADDICTED TO FOOD?

In the past the word "addiction" has been used in connection with drugs or alcohol, but when your intake of food interferes with normal healthy life, questions should be asked.

- Is food on your mind all the time?
- Do you lie about what you've eaten?
- Do you eat in secret?

- Do you eat when you're not hungry?
- Do you eat to make yourself feel better when you're not feeling good?
- Do you want to stop eating certain things, but feel you can't?
- Do you still feel cravings for certain foods after finishing a meal?
- Do you feel guilty after eating certain foods?
- Do you start making excuses for what you are eating?
- Have you tried setting rules about what you eat and failed to keep to them?

HABIT OR ADDICTION?

Throughout the book, I've talked about overeating as an addiction. It's important to be able to regard your problem in that way because all too often it is dismissed as "just a habit." We regard habits as trivial little things that we should be able to overcome with willpower. This doesn't do justice to the scale of the problem and it doesn't recognize the nature of the trap.

A habit is something we feel we control and, therefore, we should be able to stop. It's easy to see that addiction is a more serious matter that requires more than mere willpower to overcome.

You hear junk eaters dismissed as people who can't resist temptation. But does that explain how a woman can get to 200 pounds without doing anything about it? Do you really think people enjoy being obese? It's about much more than temptation.

Temptation is the desire to do something you really enjoy. No one enjoys overeating or junk eating. It makes you miserable. You wish you could stop but can't. The force that keeps you hooked is not temptation; it's addiction.

It's easy for us to recognize that a heroin addict is addicted and that willpower won't cure her. She has to see that any pleasure or crutch she thinks she gets from the drug is nothing more than the partial relief of the craving caused by withdrawal from the previous fix. The drug doesn't actually do anything for her whatsoever. It merely creates its own need.

You might not see the parallel between your predicament and that of a heroin addict, but the trap works in exactly the same way. It's not habit that makes you overeat and you won't conquer the craving through willpower. The only way to get rid of the craving permanently is to remove the cause.

THE CRAVING FOR JUNK IS CAUSED BY EATING JUNK

IN HER OWN WORDS: CHARLOTTE

I wanted to be a chemical engineer when I left school and the first university I visited told me informally they didn't take girls on engineering courses. That was my first real exposure to how the odds even in the 1990s were stacked against women, but it didn't make me give up my dream; it made me more determined to succeed.

I got a place at another, more broad-minded university,

earned my degree and landed a job immediately. I was the only woman in a department of 15 and I was regarded as something of a curiosity. I don't think the men knew how to handle it, to be honest, but I made sure I stayed strong and didn't allow any prejudice to get in my way. The work could be pretty high pressure at times, with long days and weekends too sometimes, and I took to snacking to get me through. I would always have a bag of candy on the go; then I started having a cake every day with my coffee. That became two cakes as I started craving something sweet at break time, and before long I'd put on 25 pounds!

By the time I met my husband in my late 20s, I was known as "Tubs" among all my friends and colleagues. I'd become a big cuddly lump and everybody assumed I was happy that way because I played up to it. Underneath, I was miserable as sin. When we got married, I wanted to show everybody the real me and I managed to lose 25 pounds. It took all my willpower and, as soon as that wedding dress came off, I ballooned again.

I remember looking at myself in the mirror one day and crying for ages. I could still see the face of the younger, slimmer me, but around it was this huge body, like I was wearing a fat suit. I vowed to get rid of it once and for all, and I went on another diet. It was a miserable experience, eating meagre rations of tasteless rubbish, but I stuck it out for six months, getting lots of oohs and aahhs from people who had no idea how much I was suffering. But I couldn't keep it up forever, so I caved in and, to my horror, I piled all the weight back on in a matter of weeks.

I couldn't believe my behavior around food. I was like a woman possessed! I seemed to have lost the ability to say no. I was ashamed of my weakness in the face of temptation and I became very depressed, which only made my eating worse. I was convinced that I was destined to be obese for the rest of my life, that it was my destiny because of the way I was made. But the thing that confused me was that on the one hand I was building a very good career, managing teams of men who once wouldn't have dreamed of even working alongside a woman, while on the other I was too weak to resist a candy bar.

It was only when I discovered Allen Carr's Easyway that I found the answer to my confusion. I was trying to apply my willpower to a problem that required a completely different solution. The more I tried to will myself out of it, the deeper into it I fell. When I approached the problem without using willpower, I found it so easy to change the way I ate and the pounds fell off me so fast it was incredible!

I'm so grateful to Allen Carr. He was the only one who pointed out that willpower would not help me to solve my problem. And he was the only one who was right.

It takes a strong will to persist in doing something that goes against all your instincts. When you think about the lengths you go to in order to feed your desire for junk, you couldn't do all that without being strong-willed. How do you react when people tell you that you have to eat less? Don't you find you tend to do the opposite? Wouldn't you describe that as wilful? The world is full of strong-willed people who are overweight. You don't get to the top of any industry if you're weak-willed. It takes determination, persistence, and hard work. So why would someone with the willpower to be the best in their field lack the willpower to stop eating junk? The answer is obvious:

STOPPING DOESN'T REQUIRE WILLPOWER

In fact, it tends to be the most strong-willed people who find it hardest to succeed with the willpower method, because when the door fails to open they won't give up and try to find an easier method; they'll force themselves to keep pushing on the hinges until they can push no more.

With Easyway, you arrive at your goal as soon as you remove the desire for junk and stop eating it. You remove the desire by understanding that it does nothing for you whatsoever and that there is nothing to fear about life without it. By now, you should be quite clear on both these points. As long as you believe that you're making a sacrifice, you'll never reach the end of the road.

The willpower method doesn't only make it harder to get free; it actually encourages you to stay trapped because:

- it reinforces the myth that escaping is hard and, therefore, adds to your fear.
- it creates a feeling of deprivation, which you will seek to relieve in your usual way—by eating junk.

Failing to change the way you eat using the willpower method makes it harder to try again because you'll have reinforced the belief that it's impossible to cure your problem. Some people who fail with the willpower method say they felt an enormous sense of relief when they first gave in, but that it didn't make them happy. In fact, it made them even more miserable. Anyone who tells you it's a pleasure is confusing pleasure with the relief of ending the pain. No one thinks, "Great! I've fallen back into the junk-eating trap." It's not a pleasure; it is a deeply upsetting experience, full of guilt, shame, fear, and hopelessness.

OTHER DIETERS

There will always be people who appear to succeed in losing weight by the willpower method. Their example can be damaging to your own desire to lose weight. These people tend to fall into two camps: the Braggers and the Whiners. They either brag about the sacrifices they're making or they whine about them. Both reinforce the myth that getting free from junk eating and overeating requires sacrifice.

SEVENTH INSTRUCTION: IGNORE ANY ADVICE THAT CONFLICTS WITH EASYWAY

This is important because people who claim to have lost weight by the willpower method will be very eager to give you the benefit of their wisdom. They'll be proud of the effort they've made and the fact that, to the casual observer at least, it appears to have worked. What they won't tell you is that they're still waiting for the day when they don't have to make a conscious effort any more.

People who changed their eating through willpower are always waiting for the moment when the hardship ends and they become happy and relaxed with their new diet. But with Easyway there is no need to wait. You achieve that happy state of mind the moment you remove the desire to eat junk.

Contrary to what the Braggers and Whiners may tell you, there is no sacrifice required. You're making great progress toward changing the way you eat for the better, without any need for willpower. All you've had to do is follow a simple set of instructions. You haven't been required to "give up" anything. When you understand how addiction works, you lose the fear of success. Take away the fear and you win the tug-of-war. It's easy.

The third instruction was to start off with a sense of elation. If you're still struggling to feel that thrill then you've either missed something, in which case you need to go back and reread the relevant chapter, or there's one last piece of brainwashing that is preventing you from feeling the sense of elation. Some people who try and fail to stop with the willpower method go one step further than concluding that they're weak-willed and put their failure down to another aspect of their personality over which they have no control.

When all other explanations fail them, there's one theory that conveniently provides the excuse they need to stay in the trap: the so-called addictive personality theory.

SUMMARY

- People who try to succeed with the willpower method never win the tug-of-war. They always believe they're being deprived.

- If you see your problem as just a habit, you'll assume you can conquer it with willpower. When you see it as addiction, you can begin to see the way out of the trap.

- Addiction is not a symptom of being weak willed. In fact, it's often the opposite.

- With the willpower method, you never reach your goal.

- People who brag or whine about losing weight with willpower still believe they're making a sacrifice.

- With Easyway, you reach your goal the moment you reverse the brainwashing and stop eating junk.

- Seventh instruction: IGNORE ANY ADVICE THAT CONFLICTS WITH EASYWAY.

CHAPTER 13

THE ADDICTIVE
PERSONALITY THEORY

IN THIS CHAPTER
•*A SCIENTIFIC EXCUSE* •*PERSONALITY OR MONSTER?*
•*WHY SOME PEOPLE GET MORE HOOKED THAN OTHERS*
•*A DIFFERENT BREED* •*THE EFFECT, NOT THE CAUSE*
•*EMBRACE THE TRUTH*

If you believe you were born to be a junk eater, you might feel it's futile even trying to change. In which case, why are you reading this book?

A perennial favorite topic of discussion among mothers of young children is the Nature versus Nurture debate. Do you believe that a child's personality is predetermined before they're born? Or do you think they're formed by events that take place in their early years? Mothers of more than one child will point to the personality differences between those siblings and say it's the way they were born. And each year scientists come up with new evidence of a genetic link to everything from happiness to homicide.

This is wonderful news for hopeless addicts who are suffering from the fear of success and need an excuse to stay in the trap.

If a scientist can prove that they have an addictive personality, then what's the point in trying to escape? It's out of their hands. Now they can pity themselves for being born that way, rather than despising themselves for lacking the willpower to control their eating.

We're well aware that all the other excuses we make just so that we can keep eating junk are feeble—we feel pathetic hearing ourselves say them—but the addictive personality excuse is different. It has science behind it! Who are we to doubt it?

The theory is that some people have a flaw in their genetic make-up that makes them more susceptible than most to becoming addicted. It's an attempt to explain not only why some people become addicts and others don't, but also why some addicts fall deeper into the trap than others and why they develop multiple addictions. The theory that some people are genetically programed to become addicts could explain all these phenomena, but it is no use to you for two very strong reasons:

- It doesn't solve your problem; it merely justifies it.
- There is nothing in the theory that says you can't change your personality or behavior.

The fact that you picked up this book suggests you believe you can be cured. And there is abundant evidence that our behavior can be altered by the conditions in which we're raised: discipline, principles, manners... those two siblings we mentioned may be very different in personality, but they can both be taught how to be polite.

THE GOOD NEWS FROM EASYWAY

There are many reasons why women overeat. It's not just about childhood trauma, low self-esteem, or depression. Sometimes it's as simple as the fact that food seems to taste good and is always available. That's why you have to choose what you eat carefully. The point of this book is to change your relationship with food, so that you only eat what is good for you, meaning food you will truly enjoy. The amazing thing is you won't be "giving up" anything, and your life will become better in every way.

PERSONALITY OR MONSTER?

Just as a failed attempt to lose weight will make you believe you lack the willpower to control your eating, it can also reinforce the addictive personality theory. If you put all your effort into something but still fail, it's natural to assume that it's beyond your power to resolve. The Braggers and Whiners who claim to have controlled their eating through sheer willpower also add weight to the theory. They can go months or even years maintaining their weight loss yet still crave junk! It must be their personality, right?

Wrong. They didn't crave junk food before they became hooked on it. The craving has nothing to do with their personality; it's the Big Monster, which they've failed to destroy.

If you remember, the Little Monster is the restless feeling you get when you're withdrawing from your last fix; the Big Monster is the belief that junk food gives you some sort of pleasure or crutch, and the only way to relieve the restless feeling is to consume more of it. The willpower method focuses only on killing the Little Monster. It ignores the Big Monster and, in fact, makes it stronger by encouraging the belief that you're making a sacrifice.

It's not only the Little Monster that can arouse the Big Monster; genuine hunger will also trigger it.

This can be very confusing if you quit with the willpower method. You can force yourself to go without junk for weeks and months—long enough to kill the Little Monster well and truly— yet you're still getting the cravings.

As long as you allow the Big Monster to remain alive in your head, you'll always be vulnerable to a feeling of deprivation and a craving for forbidden fruit. Braggers and Whiners kill off the Little Monster within days of changing the way they eat, but they never kill the Big Monster.

THE SO-CALLED ADDICTIVE PERSONALITY IS NOTHING MORE THAN THE BIG MONSTER AT LARGE

Killing the Big Monster is easy, provided you keep an open mind. If you choose to hide behind the excuse that you have an addictive personality, it shows that your mind is not open and you risk sentencing yourself to a lifetime of slavery.

WHY SOME PEOPLE GET MORE HOOKED THAN OTHERS

If personality is not a hindrance to escaping addiction, why do some people fall deeper into the trap than others? Why can one person eat a couple of cookies whereas another has to eat the whole package? And why is it so common for smokers, drinkers, and gamblers to have eating problems too? Doesn't that suggest that some people have a personality that's more prone to addiction than others?

Multiple addictions are caused by the same thing, but it's not your personality or your genes. It's the misguided belief that the thing you're addicted to gives you a genuine pleasure or crutch. In trying to quit one addiction, addicts will often try to substitute one drug for another; for example, a drinker might take up smoking or a smoker might start eating chocolate. The end result, more often than not, is that they become hooked on both.

Using substitutes only makes matters worse because it doesn't address the real problem: the Big Monster. On the contrary, it creates a second Little Monster. One addiction becomes two. Multiple addictions occur when you don't understand the nature of the trap you're in.

REMOVING THE DRUG IS NOT ENOUGH. YOU HAVE TO REMOVE THE DESIRE FOR THE DRUG

The Big Monster is created by conditioning and we're all conditioned differently by all sorts of things: parental guidance, peer pressure, education, neighborhood, religion, income, opportunity...

For some people, the effect of the conditioning is greater than for others because circumstances have given them a greater sense of need. All these factors have a bearing on how easily we are drawn into the trap and then how rapidly we descend.

The restrictions in our lives also control our rate of descent. Some of us are restricted by what we can afford, some by the time we have for eating, but if all the restrictions were taken out of our way, all junk food addicts would tend toward eating more, not less, because that's how addiction works.

The obesity epidemic is most severe among the wealthy nations. The people who fall deepest into the trap are the ones with the greatest opportunity, the most money, and the greatest desire because of the way they've been conditioned.

A DIFFERENT BREED

Then there are the people who don't fall into the trap at all—those lucky ones who can happily say no to a cookie. To junk eaters and overeaters, these people seem to be a different breed. They make you feel slightly uncomfortable. You feel much more at home with your fellow addicts with whom you appear to share similar character traits. To the brainwashed mind, this can look like further evidence of a shared personality defect that has led you all to overeat. But what are those personality traits that you have in common with other overeaters? An unstable temperament, which swings between exuberance and misery, a tendency toward excess, a high susceptibility to stress, evasiveness, anxiety, insecurity? These traits are all caused by addiction; they're not the reason you're addicted. Remember:

THE DESIRE FOR JUNK IS CAUSED BY EATING JUNK

People with a weight problem feel more comfortable in the company of other overeaters for one simple reason: They won't challenge you or make you think twice about your problem, because they're in the same boat. All addicts know that they're doing something illogical. If you're surrounded by other people doing the same thing, you don't feel quite so foolish.

One of the best things about getting free from overeating is that you also get free from the harmful effect it has on your whole being. You'll be able to enjoy the company of all sorts of people, overeaters or not. You just need to understand that you didn't become hooked on junk food because you have an addictive personality. If you think you have an addictive personality, it's simply because you got hooked on junk food.

THE JUMPING GENE!

The study of genetics looks for anomalies, seeking to explain why some people buck the trend. But in the case of overeating, the addiction is the trend. Are we to believe that in just a handful of decades the majority of the people in the world have suddenly been born with an addictive personality?

Let's say there was a gene that predisposed people to become addicts. It would be reasonable to assume that this gene would have appeared in a fairly constant percentage of the world population and in the same geographical concentrations throughout history. Yet this is not the case. Obesity statistics have rocketed in the last half a century. That's a minute dot on the timescale of human evolution. Smokers like to blame their addictive personality too. In the 1940s, more than 80 percent of the UK adult male population was hooked on nicotine; today it's less than 25 percent. What happened to that addictive gene?

A similar trend is evident throughout most of Western Europe and North America. At the same time, the number of smokers in Asia has soared. So has this gene hopped across from Europe into Asia?

The statistics make a mockery of the theory.

EMBRACE THE TRUTH

Your weight problem has nothing to do with your personality or genetic make-up and everything to do with the brainwashing you've been subjected to from birth. The hopelessness you feel when you can't control your eating leads you to try to blot out the problem and pretend it doesn't exist. You lie to yourself about the state you're in and laugh it off with other addicts, but deep down you know it's no laughing matter; it's a miserable situation and if you could end it with a wave of a magic wand you wouldn't hesitate. So hiding behind the theory of the addictive personality is futile. You might be able to fool other people, but you can't fool yourself.

Using any excuse just so you can carry on eating junk means consigning yourself to a lifetime of slavery and the risk of serious health problems. Think about that. Wouldn't you rather be happy? Clinging to the excuse of the addictive personality is like clinging to a lifebelt that's chained to the sinking ship.

LET GO!

Free yourself by opening your mind to the reality of your situation and the simple steps you need to take to escape it. There is a wonderful life awaiting you, free from junk food, free from denial, free from excuses and self-delusion. This is real life, the life Mother Nature designed you to enjoy, and it feels great!

If you've followed all the instructions so far, then you've already taken a big step towards freedom. You've overcome denial and accepted that you have an addiction to junk food. You've also taken action to do something about the problem. That's another big step. Now all you have to do is kill the Big Monster. Once the Big Monster is dead, you'll find it easy to cut off the supply to the Little Monster and it will die very quickly.

Remember, people who try to escape from the junk food trap

with the willpower method never kill the Big Monster; they think it's enough just to kill the Little Monster.

But you're well on your way to killing the Big Monster. You know in your heart that junk food doesn't give you pleasure or a crutch; it makes you miserable and a slave. You also understand that any feeling of pleasure that you associate with it is merely an illusion created by relieving the craving. There's no sense in continuing to eat junk just to get that relief, any more than there is in wearing tight shoes just for the relief of taking them off.

Even if you still believe that you may have been born with a predisposition to get hooked on junk, that doesn't mean you can't do something about it. Poor eyesight is linked to genetics. If you became nearsighted, would you not do something to correct it? We change our physique, personality, and behavior constantly throughout our lives in response to our role models, our environment, the obstacles that confront us, etc. We change because we're constantly in search of what's best for us—it's our instinctive quest for happiness. You know that junk food isn't good for you and that if you could stop eating it, you would be happy. So forget the addictive personality excuse and embrace the truth:

YOU CAN GET FREE JUST AS EASILY AS YOU GOT HOOKED

You have nothing to fear. The fear of living the rest of your life without eating junk is built on the illusion that junk food gives you pleasure or a crutch. To help you complete your escape, therefore, we need to make sure you can see through the illusion completely and that all remaining traces of the brainwashing are removed.

SUMMARY

- The addictive personality theory doesn't solve your problem; it merely justifies it.

- There's nothing in the theory that says you can't change your personality or behavior.

- Different people get addicted to different degrees because the conditioning is different for all of us.

- The personality traits shared by overeaters are caused by their addiction; they're not the cause.

- Accept that there's a cure for your problem and you can set about getting free.

- To get free forever, you have to kill the Big Monster.

Chapter 14

REVERSE THE BRAINWASHING

Reversing the brainwashing is easy. All you have to do is look at the foods you eat more closely and allow your senses to do their job.

The food industry is like a runaway train. It's become so vast and so powerful, with huge numbers of people depending on it for their livelihood as well as filling their shopping cart, that it would take a very brave politician to stand up to it now and order it to change its ways. The industry will claim that it performs a vital role for the benefit of humankind, but so much natural food goes to waste while millions are left starving. The problem is that the fat cats who drive the food industry have no interest in the benefit of humankind as a whole. They've found a way to fool people into paying over the odds for cheap foods that do them no good, and they have no interest in stopping the train.

In the face of such an irresistible force, you might be wondering how it can be easy for you to reverse the brainwashing. The answer is simple: forget about the food industry, forget about everybody else in the world, and focus your attention on yourself. All too easily we get swept along with the crowd, never stopping to examine how we really feel about the options that are put in front of us. As a result, we don't really make our own decisions at all; our minds are made up for us.

If you can stop and see that you've been brainwashed, you're well on your way to getting free. The next step is to make your mind up to do something about it. The final step is to do it.

EIGHTH INSTRUCTION: GO FOR IT!

This is probably the instruction you've been waiting for, but if you think it means you have to try and stop a runaway train, rest assured it does not. The challenge that lies ahead of you now is more like finding your way out of a maze. Mazes are designed to give us fun, they're not supposed to be a means of torture, so relax and enjoy the process. It won't be hard because we already know the way out and have written down the instructions for you. All you have to do is follow them. While you do, enjoy the process and take pleasure in the progress you're making. Moreover, think about the wonderful new life that awaits you when you get out.

BOX CLEVER

Research shows that women are more susceptible to

food ads on TV than men. Advertisers like to show that eating their products is a rewarding social experience and this leads to increased desire for, and consumption of, the foods they're promoting. In fact, advertisers target women when planning food ads and that's because most women hold the purse strings and the shopping list when it comes to food shopping.

A TWO-PRONGED ATTACK

As you focus on yourself and your own eating, you need to pay close attention to two things. First, concentrate on the foods that are good for you and start recognizing what wonderful and beneficial packages they are. Every time you take a knife and cut open a ripe, juicy peach, orange, pineapple, or pear, breathe in those amazing aromas, feel your mouth watering at the prospect of that delicious flavor, look at the juice glistening on the moist flesh, and relish the high content of cool, refreshing water. Every time you wash some berries and apples and grapes, appreciate the energy and nutrients that your body is going to derive from them, with barely any effort and a minimum of waste.

Second, pay closer attention to the foods that you've always believed to be your favorites. You will quickly see them for what they really are. Whenever you eat a piece of meat, imagine it in your mouth as you chew and try to discern exactly what it is you're tasting. Is there any real flavor, apart perhaps from the fruit sauce that you're eating it with? Do you really want this graying ball of flesh sliding down into your stomach, where it will sit for ages while your body pulls out all the stops to digest it and then dispose of all the toxins and waste matter? Do you really want to finish the meal feeling less energetic than when you started? You don't have to cut out meat—just stop making it the main attraction on your plate. What's wrong with a small side order of meat instead of a housebrick-sized slab surrounded by a few token vegetables?

Scrutinize all the food you eat in this way. Try it with your favorite chocolate bar. Eat it slowly, roll each mouthful around your tongue, and try to identify exactly what it is that you think you like about it. Imagine all that fat and refined sugar being chewed to a pulp before descending into your stomach. Do you really want to swallow it?

A real giveaway of bad eating is the speed with which we devour food. We claim that our favorite junk foods taste so good, and yet we can't wait to get them past our tongue and into our digestive system. That's because the taste is actually of little consequence. It's the illusion of pleasure that makes us want the food in the first place —an illusion caused by addiction to junk food.

When you take the time to really focus on the food you eat, you notice a stark contrast between the genuine enjoyment derived from eating fruit and the illusory pleasure of eating junk food. Yet this is the part that seems most difficult for many people to accept. They still fear that they'll be deprived of their favorite foods.

Smokers who try to quit using the willpower method experience a similar fear. They worry that they'll never be able to concentrate or enjoy a social occasion ever again once they no longer have cigarettes.

This is because they haven't understood that smoking didn't enhance their concentration or enjoyment of social occasions in the first place. They only thought it did because when they lit a cigarette on those occasions they temporarily relieved another problem—the withdrawal symptoms from the previous nicotine fix. People with eating problems make the same false connections. What they believe to be enjoyment and relaxation is an illusion. They confuse the temporary relief of their craving for junk food with genuine pleasure.

An interesting question arises at this point: What does it matter whether the pleasure is genuine or illusory if the person believes it? In other words, if you think you're getting pleasure, isn't that enough to make you happy?

We only need to point to the misery of millions of junk eaters to prove that this is clearly not the case. The "pleasure" they think they get from their "favorite" foods is a false pleasure that not only diminishes the more they come to depend on those foods, but also fools them into thinking they're getting a benefit when, in fact, they are doing themselves untold harm.

If you can choose between genuine pleasure and false pleasure, doesn't it make sense to pick the one that does you good?

IN HER OWN WORDS: GHISLAINE'S STORY

When I started losing weight with Easyway, just about all the food I ate was cooked and I found it hard to believe that all these cooked meals could become a thing of the past. It didn't help that I found the smell of most types of cooking absolutely gorgeous, especially bacon, curries, and bread. The thing that changed my perception was when I became aware of the effect that cooking has on food—rather than enhancing it, it destroys the nutrients. It might make inedible foods edible, but it's not how we were designed to eat. Once I got that idea into my head, it became easy to shift my diet away from cooked foods towards more fresh fruit and vegetables without feeling I was making any sacrifice at all. In fact, I would say my diet definitely became more varied and interesting.

Ghislaine's testimony is interesting because she talks about the smell of cooked foods. Many foods do indeed smell gorgeous when they're being cooked, but that's usually because we associate those smells with something we've been brainwashed into believing is a great pleasure and the ending of our hunger. Our sense of smell was given to us to enable us to track down food. When we smell food, it triggers hunger—or rather a heightened awareness of a hunger that may previously have been indiscernible. If we eat so much cooked food that it becomes the norm, we merely condition ourselves to seek out cooked food, and so the smell of cooked food will make us feel hungry. Mother Nature didn't design us to use our senses in isolation. Think about the cat approaching food: It doesn't only use its sense of smell; it uses all its senses. We have to learn to do the same. Roasted coffee and freshly lit tobacco may smell good to many young people, but their taste reveals them to be addictive drugs. Not because they taste good—quite the opposite. The kids become convinced that they could never get hooked on them because they're so disgusting. Little do they know, the trap has already been sprung. Addiction has nothing to do with taste.

We need to realize that we've been conditioned to react as we do to the smell of processed food and then do something to reverse the brainwashing. Then, like Ghislaine, we can begin to eat the foods that we know are right for us and start to cut out those that are bad without feeling that we are missing out.

WHO'S BRAINWASHING WHO?

We're trying to bring about a change in your mindset to help you see that the foods that are best for you are also the foods that taste best. You might feel that this is just another form of brainwashing; in which case let's clear up any doubts with a favourite analogy.

Imagine you've fallen in love with your dream partner. Everything about them is perfect: a handsome face, good body, sparkling personality, kindly nature. There's just one thing wrong —they don't like you.

However, you do have an admirer who thinks you're the most wonderful creature on Earth. They swoon every time they see you. To quote the song, they'd walk a million miles for one of your smiles. Sadly, you'd go to the ends of the Earth to avoid them. You can't stand them. You find them ugly, witless, and irritating and you wish they'd leave you alone.

Now a sorceress comes to you offering two pills, of which you can choose one. Both, she says, will solve your problem. The first will make you fall head over heels in love with the person who loves you. This pill costs ten pounds. The second will make the person with whom you're besotted adore you just as you adore them. This pill will cost you a thousand pounds. You can afford it. Which pill would you buy?

If you think about it, the first pill has the obvious advantages. It's much cheaper and it leaves everyone satisfied, while the second pill will leave your undesirable admirer still adoring you. Even so, most of us would choose the second pill. Why? Because we want to maintain our own sense of reality. The second pill wouldn't alter our perception of the beautiful person, whereas the first pill would be tricking us into believing something that is not true: i.e. that the ugly, witless person is beautiful and great company.

Now let's change the scenario a little. Imagine the sorceress came along before you met these two people and put one of her magic pills in your food while you weren't looking. You've swallowed the pill and it's tricked you into seeing the first person as handsome and charming and the second person as ugly and irritating, when in reality it's the other way round. So the person who adores you is really the perfect one—you just don't see it that way.

Sometimes we need a little help to see things as they really are. When it comes to food we're not given the true picture. In Chapter Five, we asked whether it had ever crossed your mind that your favorite foods were actually tasteless. Until that thought is planted in your mind, it's only natural that you'll believe all the brainwashing that has convinced you that these foods are delicious. But when you're presented with the other side of the picture, you begin to make your own judgments and quickly the scales fall from your eyes.

Provided you're willing to open your eyes and your mind, Easyway can provide the clues that will help you to see without any doubt what is real and what is an illusion.

You've been brainwashed into believing that foods such as meat, desserts, cakes, and confectionery are beautiful, but you know they don't love you. Worse than that, they're out to kill you. Meanwhile, there are foods that genuinely love you and care for you, foods that will look after you throughout your life, keeping you healthy and strong. Yet you treat these foods with disdain. You see vegetables as nothing more than an optional and quite inconvenient side order; fruit is merely an unsophisticated snack or pudding; leaves are rabbit food; nuts and grains hamster food.

This is how warped our perception becomes when we're subjected to all the brainwashing. It's time you opened your eyes and mind to the full picture, so you can decide for yourself. You will quickly see the truth:

THE FOODS THAT ARE BEST FOR YOU ARE THE ONES THAT TASTE THE BEST

LET NATURE TAKE ITS COURSE

From now on you'll find yourself analyzing all processed foods and questioning why they've been processed. Is it just to make them appear more palatable? What has it done to the nutritional value of the natural food? And how does it really taste? You're successfully reversing the brainwashing. You will be amazed at how natural and easy this feels because you're reverting to Mother Nature's plan. What could be more natural than that?

Animals don't need sell-by dates to tell them when food is no longer good to eat. They use their senses—all of them—and so can you. If only one sense rejects a food, take heed! This is especially true if something smells good but tastes bad, such as coffee. It's a combination that usually indicates an addictive drug combined with a poison. You have all the equipment an animal has to help you avoid poison, and find and enjoy your favorite food; you're just not used to using it because you've been conditioned not to. But your senses don't stop working just because you ignore them. All you have to do is pay attention to what they're telling you.

We also talk about a sixth sense; we sometimes call it intuition. It's a sense we can't pin down in the same way as the other five senses, but think about when your sixth sense comes into play. Isn't it when your logical mind is in conflict with your instinct? You look up and down the road and see no traffic, but as you go to step off the kerb, something holds you back—just as a cyclist goes by, a cyclist that you were sure wasn't there. Your sixth sense has saved you.

Sometimes we look but don't see, listen but don't hear, touch but don't feel. But if one sense fails, the others are there to step in. You didn't see the cyclist, but perhaps you heard them, though you failed to register the fact, preferring to believe your eyes. Your intellect told you it was safe to cross the road, but your senses knew it wasn't and they weren't going to give up on you that easily. After all, they're what have enabled our species to survive for millions of years. Could it be that your sixth sense is a warning sign that represents the other five senses when they're being overruled by your intellect?

Animals don't have their senses confused by intellect and they don't suffer with the eating problems that humans have. They use pure instinct as their guide—the same guide that Mother Nature provided for us. Once you understand and accept that this guide is the greatest knowledge there is on how we should eat, you'll see why Easyway is the logical solution. For the first time in your life you'll be able to approach your weight problem without feeling any confusing clash between your own brainwashed logic and your instinct. True logic and your instinct will be in perfect accord.

SUMMARY

- **Realize you've been brainwashed, make up your mind to do something about it, and go for it!**

- **It's as easy and enjoyable as escaping from a maze when you've got all the instructions.**

- **Pay closer attention to good and bad foods, so you can see them as they really are.**

- **If only one sense rejects a food, heed it.**

- **Instinct and logic do not conflict when you follow Mother Nature's Guide.**

- **Eighth instruction: GO FOR IT!**

CHAPTER 15

KNOWING WHEN TO EAT AND WHEN TO STOP

IN THIS CHAPTER

- *THE REAL REASON FOR EATING* • *MOTHER NATURE'S FUEL GAUGE*
- *HUNGER AND TASTE* • *THE NINTH INSTRUCTION*
- *READING THE GAUGE* • *WHY WE OVEREAT*
- *THE MYTH OF VARIETY* • *THE MARGIN FOR ERROR*

Mother Nature has provided an ingenious gauge that tells us when it's time to eat. Learn to read the gauge and every meal will become a pleasure.

Do you ever ask yourself why we associate eating with pleasure? The food industry will claim it's because they make their food so tasty, but, regardless of whether or not that's true, they're putting the cart before the horse. The pleasure you get when something tastes good is a function of the human body, designed to encourage you to continue seeking good things to eat.

The genuine pleasures in life come when we do things that are good for our survival: eating healthy food, quenching your thirst, playing games, socializing with friends, having sex, bathing, sleeping. Pleasure is not an optional luxury; it is a fundamental part of our ability to survive and thrive.

In Chapter 7 we began to look at the reasons why we eat. The obvious answer is that we'd die of starvation if we didn't, but that isn't what drives us to eat three square meals a day or snack between meals. The most common reasons given for eating are:

- Routine
- Temptation
- Boredom
- Restlessness
- To be sociable.

It always takes a while before anybody mentions the one true reason for eating. Eating is refueling, so what is it that prompts you to refuel your car? The need to kill time? To distract yourself from stress or boredom? To give your car a reward? It's 5 o'clock and you always refuel at 5 o'clock?

You refuel your car when the fuel gauge tells you that you're running low. Mother Nature also gave us each our own fuel gauge; the problem is we've become conditioned to ignore it. As children, we have our parents to make sure we eat and they feed us at set times each day. By the time we leave home, we've learned the routine off by heart and we know we only have to look in the fridge, or visit the supermarket or a restaurant and we can obtain food. Therefore, we tend to eat according to routine or convenience, rather than when our natural fuel gauge tells us we need food.

So what is this fuel gauge that tells you when you're running low and need to eat?

HUNGER

Hunger is the natural function that tells all animals, humans included, when they need to refuel and compels them to make the effort required to find food. In this respect it is much more ingenious than the fuel gauge on a car. Forget routine, temptation, boredom, restlessness, sociability, and all the many other reasons people give us for eating; the one true reason we eat is to satisfy hunger.

> *"Anytime you truly listen to your hunger and fullness, you lose weight."*
> **Geneen Roth, author**

A PLEASURE WORTH WAITING FOR?

When a wild animal feels hungry, it begins to look for food. This can be a long and arduous task and it could be several hours before it finds the food it needs. When humans feel hungry, we're usually able to find food within minutes. The thought of having to go hungry for a prolonged length of time concerns us. We associate hunger with starvation—in fact, we use expressions like "I'm starving" or "I'm famished" when we've gone hungry for any length of time. This is a gross exaggeration, of course. Most of us have absolutely no idea what it feels like to starve. If we did, we wouldn't use the word so lightly. Starvation is agony. What we call hunger is anything but. In fact, hunger is a sensation that contributes to the enjoyment of eating.

Satisfying your hunger is one of the greatest pleasures in life and, provided that you follow Mother Nature's Guide and all of the instructions, it's one that you can enjoy more than once a day, every day for the rest of your life.

Next time you feel hungry, try not to eat something immediately but leave it for half an hour or so and take the time to examine how it really feels. You know you're not going to suffer. Your hunger isn't doing you any harm. Your stomach might rumble, but that's hardly painful, is it? Any suffering you experience is purely psychological. If you tell yourself you're being deprived, you'll feel miserable and you'll regard hunger as a source of misery. This is why diets are so gruelling and ultimately unsuccessful. Every time you feel hungry the sense of deprivation increases and the more miserable you feel.

We're not asking you to deprive yourself when you feel hungry. Don't worry, you'll get to eat in good time and the food will taste better than usual. The aim is for you to see hunger in a different light: Not as a threat that needs to be dealt with right away, but as a source of pleasure that will increase the longer you leave it.

The French are renowned food lovers and they devote a lot of time to the pleasure of eating. Before a meal they wish each other "Bon appetit," for the simple reason that the greater your appetite, the more you'll enjoy the meal. Another ingenious aspect of Mother Nature's plan is that food tastes better the hungrier you are.

No doubt you've experienced this for yourself. If you've ever gorged yourself on your favorite food, you'll know that the flavor diminishes after those first few mouthfuls and the more you eat, the more tasteless the food becomes until it actually ends up being repulsive.

Satisfying your hunger is one of the genuine pleasures in life that I talked about at the beginning of the chapter. In order to get the full pleasure from eating, you need to be genuinely hungry. In fact, when you're really hungry you'll find all sorts of foods pleasurable. In normal circumstances you probably wouldn't dream of eating a witchetty grub, but if you'd been walking across the Australian outback for days without food, you'd gobble up the first witchetty grub you could find and consider it a delicacy.

We're not advocating that you eat witchetty grubs, or that you deliberately deprive yourself of food just to get more pleasure from eating; the point is that if you eat when you're not hungry, you won't get the pleasure you're hoping for.

NINTH INSTRUCTION: AVOID EATING UNLESS YOU'RE HUNGRY

This is not the same as depriving yourself. You only feel deprived if you believe you're making a sacrifice. When you embrace your hunger, you're not sacrificing anything. Perhaps you think prolonging your hunger just to enhance the pleasure of eating is no different to wearing tight shoes just to feel the relief of taking them off. Wearing tight shoes is very uncomfortable, whereas hunger is not. Yet satisfying hunger is every bit as pleasurable as taking off tight shoes. Mother Nature's plan is designed to give us all the pleasure and none of the pain.

Remember, pleasure is a vital function in our ability to survive. It's a sign that we're looking after ourselves properly. If you find that you're not enjoying life and that eating is not a source of pleasure, it's because you've strayed from Mother Nature's plan. All you have to do is revert to the plan.

RESPONDING TO MOTHER NATURE'S FUEL GAUGE

Hunger indicates your need to eat just as the fuel gauge indicates your car's need for fuel. You don't stop to refuel your car as soon as the needle drops below full; you wait until the gauge is getting somewhere near empty. With Mother Nature's fuel gauge, the same principle applies.

I've already explained that the longer you go hungry, the better the food will taste and the more pleasure you'll get from eating. Learn to read your fuel gauge and you'll be able to derive maximum pleasure from every meal.

Picture hunger as a fuel

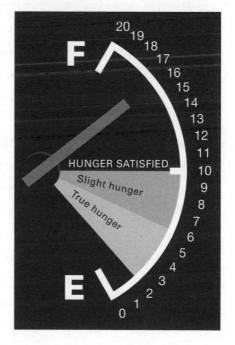

gauge numbered from 0 to 20, where 0 is empty and 20 is full up. The range between 7 and 10 is slight hunger, between 3 and 7 is true hunger, and 10 is the point at which hunger is satisfied. If you eat when the gauge is reading between 10 and 20, then you're not responding to hunger. More likely you've been tempted by a smell or some other association that has triggered a craving.

You begin to feel hungry when the gauge drops below 10, but this is only the early sensation of hunger. You can live with this feeling very comfortably. It isn't painful at all and if you embrace it, rather than regard it as a problem that you need to tackle immediately, then it will be a source of pleasure. If you eat in this zone on the gauge, you won't get the full pleasure from the food because your taste buds are not as responsive as they could be. When the needle drops below 7 into the true hunger zone, that's when you should be looking to eat.

It's important that you learn to read your fuel gauge and familiarize yourself with your own hunger so you can respond at the right time. You need to know that slight hunger can be made to feel like true hunger by factors such as the smell or sight of food. If you feel slight hunger and somebody starts talking to you about the lovely meal they ate in a restaurant the previous evening, it will make you feel hungrier than you really are. This is one of the food industry's chief weapons in brainwashing you to eat more than you really want or need. They know that if they can put their food in front of you in some shape or form, you'll think you're hungry and will feel more inclined to want it.

Recognizing the varying degrees of your own hunger is key to solving your weight problem. It's just as easy to reverse the food industry brainwashing and see that what you think is true hunger may only be slight hunger. If you can focus on something else, it may disappear completely. If you do feel it, don't panic! See it as a sign that you're heading towards another enjoyable meal and take pleasure in feeling it grow, knowing that the more it grows, the better the meal will taste.

Allowing your hunger to grow is not the same as depriving yourself. You're not denying yourself food; you're just deferring the moment of satisfaction. By doing this you're giving yourself a chance to ask yourself how hungry you really are and what food you really want to eat.

When we seek to satisfy hunger immediately, we tend to go for so-called convenience foods—processed, packaged junk that gives us barely any nutritional value whatsoever and thus fails to truly satisfy our hunger.

Which brings us on to the second part of the refueling process.

KNOWING WHEN TO STOP

When you refuel a car, the common tendency is either to keep filling until the tank is full or to put in fuel to a certain value. Both have their own merits, but neither guarantees the best performance from your car. The more fuel you put in, the heavier the car becomes and, therefore, the less efficient it is to run. In Formula One racing, they make careful calculations to make sure the cars are carrying exactly the right amount of fuel to get them to the finish line and no more.

Fortunately, we don't have to make any such calculation when we refuel—Mother Nature's fuel gauge does it for us. But again, we have to take heed.

If you start eating when the gauge is between 3 and 7, the food will taste its best. As you fill up, your hunger will abate until you reach 10, at which point your hunger is satisfied. If you

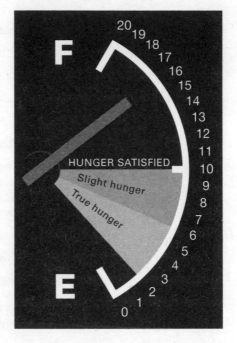

keep eating until the gauge reaches 20, you'll be completely full up. Eating beyond the point of satisfaction is what gives us that bloated, uncomfortable feeling that can leave a bad taste in the mouth—literally.

As we grow up, we're conditioned to disregard our fuel gauge. We're given a plateful of food at a fixed time of day and told to leave a clean plate, regardless of how hungry we are. And so we become accustomed to eating according to routine and custom, rather than listening to our own body's needs. But this conditioning is also easy to reverse. Having embraced hunger as the ingenious gauge that tells you when to start eating, you can then start to recognize the signals that tell you when to stop.

> **GIVE IT TIME**
>
> Eat slowly to give your body time to register that it's received the nutrients it requires. If you bolt the food down, you'll still be feeling hungry when you've eaten enough to satisfy your hunger, and you'll end up overeating.

WHY WE OVEREAT

Your hunger is satisfied once you've taken in the nutrients your body needs. Thirst works in exactly the same way, but when you drink a glass of water, you stop when your thirst is quenched, not when your belly is full. Why doesn't the same apply to eating?

The fact is it does, but only if you eat the right foods. If the food doesn't contain the nutrients your body requires, the gauge won't register "satisfied" and the only thing that will stop you eating is when you're full and can physically take no more. When you regularly eat foods with little or no nutritional value, overeating becomes the norm. This is a crucial point to remember in your quest to lose weight:

LACK OF NUTRIENTS LEADS TO OVEREATING

Only by eating the right foods will you achieve a feeling of satisfaction. And only by achieving satisfaction will you know when to stop eating. But first you have to reverse the brainwashing that has prevented you from recognizing your favorite foods and knowing when you've eaten enough.

The principle for knowing when to eat and when to stop eating is very simple: eat when you're hungry and stop when you're satisfied. Stick to this principle and you'll find that every meal becomes enjoyable and you'll have no weight problems.

THE SPICE OF LIFE

The quickest and most efficient way to satisfy your hunger is to eat foods that are packed with the nutrients you need. You might be wondering where this leaves variety. After all, you know that most of the foods available offer little or no nutritional value whatsoever.

We like to think we have varied tastes. The supermarkets don't just offer us all sorts of different types of foods, but they offer us different brands within each category, giving us the impression of choice between items that are essentially the same in all but the packaging. We're enchanted by the range of options available to us, but how much of that variety do you actually eat?

Next time you go to the supermarket, count the number of different foods in your basket. Now think how often you change the items on your shopping list. There may be the odd change from week to week, depending on the weather, or your mood, or your budget, but the majority of items will be the same week in, week out.

The cereal aisle is a case in point. You'll find a vast array of breakfast products in all sorts of different shapes and sizes, yet most of us reach for the same one or two every time. It doesn't bother us that we're not sampling all the different cereals on offer. We'll happily eat the same one every day for months, even years on end. If we ever do get the urge for a change, we'll pick a new cereal and that will become our regular for a similar length of time.

ONCE WE'VE DECIDED ON A FAVORITE FOOD, WE'RE HAPPY TO EAT IT TIME AFTER TIME

The curry house or Chinese restaurant are two more classic examples of the illusion of variety. Those menus they present us with are vast and we love to pore over them, discussing the relative merits of each dish before making our selection. And then we'll choose the dish that we know we like—the same one we always have.

So much for variety.

The fact is, we're quite happy to eat the same food meal after meal if it's our favorite food. And there's nothing wrong with that, as long as it provides the energy and nutrients that your body requires. If you think that sounds boring, don't worry. Nobody is forcing you to eat the same food day after day. You can try something new any time you like. But once it becomes one of your favorites, human nature dictates that you will try to eat it on a regular basis. After all, why wouldn't you? Given a choice between your favorite food and some other option, who in their right mind would choose the alternative?

The food industry brainwashes us into believing that we need a wide variety of foods in our diet because they want to sell as many different products as they can. Just as the concept of fashion is vital to the clothing industry, to keep people buying new clothes before the old ones have worn out, new brands are vital to the food industry to keep us buying more food than we actually need.

Just like fashion, tastes in food come and go according to a variety of factors. Shrimp cocktail and Black Forest gateau were fashionable favorites in the 1970s; today they are as outmoded as wing collars and platform shoes. But natural foods stand the test of time. Do you ever grow tired of the taste of apples?

THE MARGIN FOR ERROR

Breakfast cereals contain little or no nutritional value and, when you analyse the difference between all those varieties, you quickly come to the conclusion that they're nearly all the same: a product of wheat or corn, cooked and reshaped and virtually tasteless. What keeps us coming back for more is the high sugar content to which we get addicted.

It's a peculiar choice for your first meal of the day, when your need for nutrients is particularly high, but the food industry has been ingenious in selling us these products as "the perfect start to the day." Many people say that breakfast is their favorite meal of the day, but it's not because those cereals are so delicious or healthy. They are the very opposite. The reason we like breakfast so much is because we've gone without food all night and our taste buds are, therefore, ready to enjoy just about anything.

In Chapter 8, I explained about the Junk Margin—one of the many wonders of Mother Nature's plan, which enables all animals, including humans, to move on to secondary and tertiary foods when their favorite foods aren't available. The gorilla, for example, prefers to feed on fruit, but when fruit is not available it will eat other vegetation to survive. It doesn't make a conscious decision to force down some other vegetation to keep itself alive; it is guided by instinct. As the gorilla grows hungrier, so its second- and third-tier foods taste better and better. The gorilla doesn't have to make any conscious decision. Its hunger and taste buds make the decision for it.

But here's the vital difference between the gorilla and most of humankind: When fruit becomes available again the gorilla will revert to a fruit diet, because fruit is its favorite food—the food that tastes best to the gorilla. It has not been brainwashed into thinking otherwise.

Mother Nature has provided us with a liberal margin for error, which means that you can go on eating a fair amount of secondary foods. This Junk Margin is very important to Easyway because, unlike special diets, you never have to say, "I'm not allowed to eat this or that." There are no rigid restrictions. Remember—it isn't a JUNK FOOD MARGIN—you're going to put all that behind you. It's a Junk Margin. You can continue to eat meat, pasta, bread—all the things you eat now—provided the vast bulk of what you eat is the correct food according to Mother Nature's Guide.

People's weight problems can be explained by one simple fact: Thanks to our intelligence and the ability it gives us to spread misinformation, our Junk Margin has become the norm and the foods that were designed to be our favorites have become secondary. Your objective now is to use your intelligence to reverse that process by changing the way you perceive highly nutritious foods and how you perceive junk foods. So let's begin by agreeing on what are the right foods and what falls into the margin.

SUMMARY

- **Hunger is the one true reason for eating.**
- **See hunger as a pleasure, not a pain.**
- **Any suffering you experience when hungry is purely psychological.**
- **The hungrier you are, the better food will taste.**
- **The true pleasure to be derived from eating is the satisfying of hunger.**
- **Ninth instruction: AVOID EATING UNLESS YOU'RE HUNGRY.**
- **Stop eating when your hunger is satisfied, not when you're full.**
- **Hunger is only satisfied by eating nutritious foods.**
- **A lack of nutrients leads to overeating.**
- **Eat slowly to give the nutrients time to register.**
- **The need for variety in your diet is an illusion.**
- **Understand the purpose of the Junk Margin.**

CHAPTER 16

STAPLES OF THE JUNK MARGIN

IN THIS CHAPTER
- *SUGAR ADDICTION*
- *THE TRUTH ABOUT MEAT AND DAIRY*
- *CHANGING AS YOU GO*

Three types of food make up a major part of our regular diet. By understanding the effect of these foods and putting them in the Junk Margin, you'll easily make the change you need to the way you eat.

Given that sweet, juicy fruit is the favorite food for humans, isn't it a shame that so many of the foods that are bad for us are also sweet? You might think it would have been better if we'd been designed to eat bitter foods, then we wouldn't be so attracted to cakes, candy, and sugary drinks. But it's no coincidence that so much junk food is sweet: the food industry designed it that way to replicate the taste of our favorite food.

It's no secret that refined sugar is bad for us. We're under no illusions about that fact. Yet we find it incredibly hard to cut it out of our diet. The fact is that sugar hooks us in the same way that an addictive drug like nicotine does.

The process of refining sugar is very similar to the way the coca plant is refined into cocaine, or poppy seeds refined into heroin. Starting with a sugarcane plant, the refining strips away its fiber, vitamins, and minerals, leaving behind a white, crystalline substance that is very sweet and soluble and can be added easily to other foods to give us a similar sensory sensation to that of eating fruit. But refined sugar gives us none of the goodness of fruit. It is what's known as an "empty carb," which means it contains barely any nutritional value but is high in carbohydrate. Eating too much of it means the body taking in an excess of carbohydrate—more than it can burn—and this excess is turned into fat. But because it contains no nutritional value, it doesn't satisfy hunger, and so it creates a need to eat more. The tendency is to eat more sugar because that white, crystalline substance is also highly addictive. It also has a disastrous effect on your blood sugar level, creating false highs and causing it to crash.

To make matters worse, refined sugar is usually mixed with other processed foods, such as fat or flour, which compound the problem of putting on weight. These are not foods that we savor; they're foods that we tend to bolt down. Why? Because our only reason for eating them is to get at the drug as quickly as possible.

You can see how refined sugar has become the most harmful substance in the developed world. Heroin and cocaine addicts are relatively rare. Sugar addiction afflicts almost everyone at one time or another. Perhaps you think you're not addicted to sugar. Check the labels on every item of food you buy and then try leaving everything that contains sugar out of your diet. You'll notice a craving. It's the same craving that smokers experience between cigarettes. In this case, it's caused by the withdrawal from sugar.

If you try this exercise, you may be surprised by the number of foods that contain refined sugar. Even savory dishes that you don't associate with sweetness, such as pizzas and bags of chips, contain significant levels of sugar. That's why they're so popular. It's the sugar that fools us into thinking they're delicious.

Our love of sweet things shouldn't be seen as a weakness. It's what helped us to survive for millions of years. It was only when we decided to try and outsmart nature by creating a substance that deceived our taste buds that the love of sweetness became a problem. Now we grow up believing that sugary foods taste delicious, when in fact that delicious taste is invariably the flavor of fruit. We're also told that sugary foods will make us happy.

It's this brainwashing that creates the Big Monster in your brain. Unlike the Little Monster that cries out feebly when you're not feeding it refined sugar, the Big Monster really can make you miserable. When it's aroused, it fills your head with the feeling that you're being deprived until you get your next fix of sugar.

You need to be aware that if you eat anything that contains refined sugar you're making yourself vulnerable to becoming a sugar addict. You eat sugar for no other reason than that you've been brainwashed into believing that it gives you some sort of pleasure or crutch. The only pleasure you get from it is the temporary relief of keeping the Little Monster quiet. But if you can reverse the brainwashing and see that sugar does absolutely nothing for you whatsoever, then it's easy to kill the Little Monster and free yourself from your desire for sugar.

THE TRUTH ABOUT MEAT AND DAIRY

We all know that sugar is not good for us, but we continue to eat it because we've been brainwashed into believing it gives us pleasure or a crutch. But there are two other foods groups over which there is much more confusion:

- Meat, by which we mean the flesh of all animals, including seafood
- Dairy, by which we mean milk and all its by-products.

No only are we encouraged to eat these foods, we're told that they're essential for a healthy diet. I've already exploded the myths that we need to eat meat for protein and dairy for calcium, and talked about the relative difficulty your digestive system has in dealing with these foods. So why have they become fundamental to the human lifestyle?

When food is scarce, nature enables us to adapt to secondary foods. This is most likely how we came to eat meat in the first place, and from these extreme circumstances the whole meat industry has grown. But it's an industry about which we're utterly ashamed. How many of us would be happy to watch our next meal being slaughtered at the abattoir, or go out and kill it ourselves? We prefer to keep the killing out of our lives. Does that suggest that we're naturally inclined to eat meat?

A cat shows no such reservation when it pounces on a baby

bird. When we watch nature programs showing lions killing an antelope, we want the antelope to get away. Is that the behavior of a creature designed by nature to kill and devour meat?

Our love of animals makes it very uncomfortable for us to face the gory reality of eating meat. In fact, we're far more naturally inclined to protect animals than to kill them. Why would Mother Nature give us the emotional desire to protect something but the physical need to eat it?

Quite simply, she hasn't. The truth is we're not designed to eat meat. Compare your teeth and fingernails to the teeth and claws of even a domestic cat—do you really think you have what it takes to kill and dissect an animal with your bare hands and teeth? If you tried, you'd find you couldn't even chew the raw meat properly. If you did manage to force some down your throat, your digestive system would have to work overtime.

The stomach of a carnivore contains much more hydrochloric acid than the human stomach. This is what enables it to break meat down efficiently and its relatively short intestines enable it to dispose of the waste quickly. But the human stomach doesn't have the necessary enzymes for digesting meat efficiently, so a large amount is passed out as waste, taking as long as 20 hours for the putrifying mass to pass through your intestines.

You can imagine the wear and tear this has on your body, but we only pay it any attention when we feel the pain, in the form of indigestion, constipation, or other digestive ailments. The rest of the time it's a case of "out of sight, out of mind." Your body is much more resilient than the engine of a car and it fights hard against the abuse, but cutting up meat and feeding it into your stomach to get protein is like cutting up a plastic bucket and feeding it into your gas tank to get gasoline. Nothing is gained and all sorts of problems are caused.

So the less meat you eat, the better. This doesn't mean you have to become a vegan. You can still eat meat and fish if you want to as long as it doesn't form the basis of your diet. We've been conditioned to regard three meals a day, at least two of which and often all three contain meat, as normal and well suited to our physical needs. But when you look at it closely and see how ill equipped we are, both physically and emotionally, to eat meat, it's hard to imagine a food LESS suitable for human consumption.

Dairy, on the other hand, does not go against our love of animals. In fact, it gives us the opportunity to channel that fondness into rearing cattle and keeping them alive and healthy for as long as possible, so that they can yield the maximum volume of milk. And isn't milk the very life source that nourishes us from the day we're born?

Milk is the favorite food of all new-born mammals. It flows naturally from their mothers' breasts and provides all the vitamins and nutrients they need. We instinctively accept this as fact. When we see a baby suckling on its mother's breast, we make no attempt to vary its diet, or complement it with vitamin supplements. We're able to refer to the one section of Mother Nature's Guide that has not been torn up and recognize that the baby is getting the exact food package that was designed for it. We feel the same instinctive sense of wellbeing when we see any animal suckling its mother, be it a calf, a fawn, a puppy, or whatever.

As children we're encouraged to drink milk to help us build strong bones and teeth. But this involves a leap in logic that we take for granted. As babies we drink our mother's milk, the milk designed for us by Mother Nature. It's not the same as the milk a puppy gets, or a fawn, or a calf. The milk of all mammals is specially formulated with the specific balance of vitamins, iron, calcium, etc. that the specific infant requires. You wouldn't give a new-born baby cow's milk. But once we're weaned off our mother's milk, we're suddenly expected to drink cow's milk. It used to be compulsory drinking in British schools! Every British person of a certain age remembers those half-pint bottles of warm, sour milk on a summer's day, with half an inch of curdled cream floating at the top. This, they were told, was for their benefit!

A substance in milk called "casein" clumps together in your stomach into dense, tough curds that are hard to digest. All milk contains casein, but there is 300 times as much casein in cow's milk as there is in human milk. Just because dairy is slightly easier to consume than meat, is that reason enough to assume it's good for you? Your body does its best to cushion you from the blows, so for the most part you remain blissfully unaware of the damage being caused inside you, but if you could see it you'd think twice about dairy produce.

So should we all be drinking human milk throughout our lives? Not at all. Can you think of any animals that continue drinking milk in adulthood, other than humans and domestic pets? Milk is designed for babies, to make it easy for them to take in the diet they need for a healthy start in life. Mother Nature also designed it, so that all mammals should be weaned off milk when still young.

In order to digest milk, we need the enzymes renin and lactase. These have virtually disappeared from our digestive system by the time we reach the age of three. By this stage, we should have been weaned off milk, on to solids. If you go on drinking milk beyond this stage in life, you put a great strain on your digestive system.

CHANGE AS YOU GO

The obvious conclusion is that adults were not designed to drink milk, and certainly not the milk of another animal. It's also unnatural, both physically and emotionally, for humans to eat meat regularly. Meat and dairy are second- and third-rate foods. They're not our favorites. Our favorites are fresh fruit, nuts, vegetables, and seeds.

If you're struggling to imagine life without meat or fish, milk or cheese, you don't have to. No one's telling you to give them up. But hopefully you've read enough to at least make you question what you've been led to believe about these foods until now and to see the argument for reducing your intake of these foods.

The fact is that fresh fruit, nuts, vegetables, and seeds form a large part of most people's diet anyway, in some shape or form. You're not being asked to make radical changes, merely to tip the balance to make these foods the basis of your regular diet and put secondary foods in your Junk Margin. Your diet will be just as varied, if not more so. Your meals will taste better. And you will finish every meal feeling satisfied and reenergized.

As this way of eating becomes the norm, you'll also change your perception of the foods that you might currently think you're going to miss. Your desire for them will diminish and may disappear completely. You'll realize that the pleasure you thought you derived from them was an illusion and you'll be amazed how easily you've changed your whole way of eating.

Remember our claim: "You'll be able to eat as much of your favorite foods as you want, whenever you want." So what does Mother Nature's larder have in store?

SUMMARY

- Refined sugar is designed to replicate the sweetness we derive from fresh fruit.

- It's an "empty carb," giving you calories without any nutritional benefit.

- Sugar is also addictive, creating its own craving, which can only be satisfied by eating more sugar.

- Humans are ill equipped physically and emotionally to kill animals for food.

- Meat takes a heavy toll on the human digestive system and gives very little taste or nutritional value.

- We're only designed to drink milk as babies, and then only our mother's milk.

Chapter 17

OUR REAL FAVORITE FOODS

We've established the foods to avoid; now for the foods you can look forward to with relish.

In order to establish the food packages that were designed for human consumption by the ingenious force that created us, we need to look back to a time before we discovered the secret of fire and started cooking, planting crops, or rearing livestock. An easy way to do this is to look at the behavior of the animals that most closely resemble us. The chimpanzee shares 98 percent of our DNA and, like us, is an omnivore—it eats both vegetation and meat. But the chimp's favorite food by far is fruit, followed by leaves, accounting for around 60 percent and 25 percent of their feeding time respectively. They spend around 10 percent of their feeding time eating seeds and blossoms and only about five percent eating meat and insects.

You may have seen those incredible documentaries showing

chimpanzees hunting, killing, and eating other animals and concluded that they—and, therefore, we—are naturally disposed to eating meat. But chimpanzee experts will tell you otherwise. They've found that chimps use meat as a social tool, mostly the males, who'll distribute it among friends and deny it to enemies. They'll also offer it to females with whom they wish to mate. You might interpret this to mean that meat is a delicacy in the chimpanzee world, but what they're actually doing is using a kill to show their prowess, just as a matador kills a bull to show his courage and skill. They're not driven by a desire to eat meat. If they were, they'd be doing it all the time.

Chimpanzees find it very quick and easy to gather fruit and eat it when it's available. That's one of the beauties of fruit: you don't have to chase it and it doesn't fight back! So for that five percent of the time that chimps spend on obtaining and eating meat, they're actually getting a much poorer return than for the 60 percent they spend on fruit, meaning the actual quantity of meat they consume is even less than five percent of their diet.

A chimpanzee would much rather eat fruit and leaves. A recipe for a dull life? Hardly. Chimps have been found to feast on as many as 300 different types of plant. When was the last time you put 300 different items in your shopping basket?

Chimpanzees are stronger and faster than humans, they have boundless energy, and they don't suffer with weight problems or any of the eating disorders that have come to blight mankind. For an animal that is so closely related to us anatomically, doesn't that make you think? Nobody questions whether the chimp is getting enough variety from its diet, or whether it's getting the necessary vitamins and minerals. There is no clearer indication of Mother Nature's Guide. The chimpanzee is surrounded by food options. It has the intelligence to hunt and kill. It can make tools to "fish" for termites. But the chimpanzee has not been brainwashed into believing that these are its favorite foods. They form a tiny proportion of its diet. The food chimpanzees prefer to eat is fruit. And when you look at the evidence, it's clear that fruit is what we prefer to eat too.

NATURE'S VARIETY SHOW

I've talked about the variety of foods on sale in the supermarkets and how much of this variety is an illusion, made up of different brands of the same thing. But when you get to the fresh food section the variety is no illusion. There is an abundance of different foods, each with its own look, smell, texture, and taste, each of which can be eaten uncooked. By contrast, the range of meat and dairy products is relatively small. It shows how little effect cutting out meat and dairy will have on the variety in your diet.

Fruit	Vegetables	Seeds & nuts	Meat	Dairy
Apple	Lettuce	Brazil nut	Beef	Milk
Pear	Arugula	Walnut	Lamb	Cream
Peach	Spinach	Almond	Pork	Cheese
Banana	Cabbage	Hazelnut	Chicken	Yogurt

Pineapple	Basil	Pecan	Turkey	Butter
Plum	Coriander	Chestnut	Duck	
Orange	Parsley	Peanut	Goose	
Grape	Carrot	Sunflower seeds		
Satsuma	Celery	Sesame seeds		
Tangerine	Peas			
Clementine	Tomato			
Melon	Pepper			
Mango	Green onion			
Apricot	Bean sprouts			
Cherry	Mange-tout			
Kiwi				
Pomegranate				
Strawberry				
Raspberry				
Blackberry				
Blueberry				
Black currant				
Red currant				
Gooseberry				
Olive				

THE JUICY BIT

Fruit meets all the criteria in Mother Nature's Guide. It looks good, smells good, feels good, and tastes good. We love the flavor of fruit so much that we've learned how to extract it and add it to other things. All those puddings, cakes and confectionery that you regard as irresistible—how good would they taste without flavoring? But would they taste good if they were flavored with chicken, beef, or lamb? Can you imagine taking a bite of a cream cake that tasted of beef? Revolting! We give taste to these otherwise bland foods by adding lemon, orange, strawberry, blueberry, cherry, vanilla, almond, and so on—flavors extracted from fruits, nuts, and seeds.

If cooking meat gives it real flavor, why the need to add seasoning and sauces? Have you ever felt an apple could do with a pinch of salt? Does a banana taste better if you add garlic? Fruit requires no added flavoring. Quite the reverse; it is fruit and other plants that we add to bland foods like meat to make them palatable: applesauce with pork, cranberry sauce with turkey, mintsauce with lamb, horseradish and mustard with beef, sage and onion with chicken, etc. In some cases, the sole purpose of eating the meat is to get the flavor of the added sauce. Take snails and mussels, for example. Remove the garlic sauce and all you're left with is a mouthful of chewy flesh.

Think about our favorite drink flavours: orange, lemon, lime, strawberry, raspberry, apple, peach, pineapple, banana. And not just soft drinks either. In addition to the grapes and hops that go into wine and beer, we flavor spirits with juniper, sloe, orange, lemon, cherry, apricot, and more. We don't flavor them with meat or cheese. That would be repulsive.

So it's clear that we must have been hoodwinked somewhere along the line if we think that meat and cheese are among our favorite foods. Clearly fruit appeals to our natural instincts more than any other type of food and by now you will understand why. Taste is closely associated with hunger, and hunger is your body's way of telling you that it needs certain nutrients. Fruit provides those nutrients. Mother Nature has given us a taste for fruit to insure that we keep eating it. When we ignore that instinct, that's when things go wrong.

Fruit is the best friend your digestive system could wish for. It requires barely any breaking down, passing very quickly from the stomach to the intestines where the goodness is extracted. Water is our most vital nutrient, aiding digestion, assimilating nutrients, and disposing of waste. Fruit contains an abundance of water, some being made up of 90 percent water. And it's easy to carry around!

In fact, the more you look at the design of fruit, the more you realize how ingenious it is. Whether it's a banana, which comes in its own natural wrapper, or an apple that stays firm and shiny for weeks, always ready to eat, the Earth is brimming with an abundance of fruit that Mother Nature has presented to us in an attractive and convenient package. And every one of them has its own distinct flavor.

On hot days, fruit remains cool and refreshing. It enables us to satisfy both our hunger and our thirst at the same time. Making up the rest of the package are the minerals and vitamins that we need to stay healthy and strong. There is very little waste when we digest fruit, and what there is is easily disposed of. In stark contrast to meat, you gain far more energy from eating fruit than you use up digesting it. And you can't have too much energy. Energy is the source of human happiness. The more you have, the better you feel.

Before we become conditioned by our parents and other influences, we show very similar tastes to the chimpanzee. Babies begin life wanting only their mother's milk, but when the time comes to move off nature's liquid diet and on to solids, they turn unquestioningly to fruit. The babyfood manufacturers have come up with all sorts of concoctions to sell in those little jars that adorn the supermarket shelves, but it's always the pureed fruit that babies eat most readily. The ones containing chicken and other meats are an acquired taste.

WHY AM I HAVING TO TELL YOU THIS?

Fresh fruit is the ideal food package for humans, closely followed by fresh vegetables, nuts, and seeds. These foods provide us with all the nutrients we require. We've spent the vast majority of our time on the planet eating these foods as our staple diet. Eating processed food is a very recent phenomenon—and so is the increase in eating disorders and dietary health problems.

Two of the major concerns of modern society, health and finances, could be helped significantly by getting back to the diet that Mother Nature designed for us. Fresh fruit, supplemented by vegetables, nuts, and seeds, provides us with energy, vitamins, minerals, fiber, and water. It's easy to digest and its wastes are minimal and easy to dispose of. The varieties are endless and it is also the best value food there is. An apple is much cheaper than a chocolate bar and infinitely more satisfying. You can even grow it for free!

And yet there remains a tremendous resistance to making these foods our staple diet.

Why are the advertising billboards not showing us images of fresh fruit? Why isn't children's television peppered with ads for nuts and vegetables? Quite simply because the food industry would shrink beyond recognition if it stuck to what's good for us. It has not grown so huge by harvesting crops and selling them in their natural state. That's a tiny part of the market. The real money lies in finding ways to tamper with those crops, to process them beyond recognition and present them in new and unusual ways, to make consumers believe they're getting variety and nutrition when all they're really getting is second-rate food and a whole lot of eating problems.

It's a highly lucrative con and nobody is going to put a stop to it any time soon. Certainly not the authorities, who are supposed to be responsible for our best interests. They're utterly incapable of making up their minds about what's good for us and what's bad; they send out so many mixed messages that we don't know where to turn for the truth. Even when they do get it right, they don't go far enough. The warnings about red meat and full-fat milk are long overdue, but what do they recommend instead? Chicken and skimmed milk. They might as well be telling us to cut down on the arsenic.

Human history has been shaped by the pursuit of food. New lands have been discovered, wars have been fought, and boundaries marked out. We've literally gone to the ends of the Earth to bring back ideas and ingredients that would make our mouths water. Thousands of recipes have been concocted, thousands of books have been sold teaching the secrets of cooking, and no doubt those pioneers, merchants, chefs, and publishers all believed they were playing a part in enhancing our quality of life, but all they actually achieved was to persuade us to accept second best, by gradually perfecting the art of dressing up junk food to resemble the real thing.

We've come a long way down the wrong track and that can be hard to accept. It requires courage and imagination to accept that what appears to be an intelligent course of action is, in fact, a big mistake. But in the entire history of the human race our departure from Mother Nature's Guide is only a very recent development. For most of our time on Earth, we've lived and thrived by one simple law: Only eat food in its natural state.

A FRUITLESS EXERCISE

Our natural instincts were formed over millions of years and it doesn't take much to bring them to the fore again. You just need to learn to recognize them and to do that you must understand how processing foods affects it.

- It kills the nutrients.
- It adds toxins.
- It diminishes the water content.

One glass of water is usually enough to quench your thirst. Water is what your body is crying out for when it sends the message that it's thirsty. Try to drink another glass of water and you'll find it becomes more difficult. But try quenching your thirst with a glass of beer and you find you can drink two or three glasses and still want more. The alcohol in the beer causes dehydration —the very opposite of what you were trying to achieve—and so you continue to feel thirsty.

The same principle applies to hunger and eating: unless you provide your body with the nutrients it needs, it will continue to send the message that it's hungry.

Cooking your food in water or some other liquid will not counteract the loss of water from the food itself. Neither will drinking with the meal make up the difference. Remember the Plastic Bucket Syndrome—your digestive system is an incredibly sophisticated machine that can take in various different fuels at once, extract what it needs from each, distribute these nutrients to where they're needed, and dispose of the waste, but it only performs efficiently with the right food packages.

Food that's lost its high water content is difficult to digest and drinking can make the problem worse by flushing away the digestive juices from your stomach. While your body may keep functioning, it will not be able to dispose of all the waste as nature intended. Instead it will store it where it can, and that's where the unsightly bulges appear.

The key point to remember is that hunger is not your body crying for food; it's your body crying out for specific nutrients. We all experience different cravings from time to time. Pregnant women are known for having extreme cravings, which can seem completely fanciful. In fact, they're entirely logical. In pregnancy, the body requires extra nutrients to sustain the baby as well as the mother and the cravings are very distinct messages, calling for very specific foods.

In Chapter 15, I explained why food tastes best when you're hungry. It begs the question: Why do people continue to eat when they've gorged themselves? With all that food inside them, they can't be hungry any more, so surely they're still craving the food for its taste.

If you've been in this situation, you'll know that this is not the case. When you're full up, the food starts to taste bland or even sickly, and yet you still have the desire to eat. The reason is actually very simple: You ARE still hungry. Until you learn what hunger really is, it's hard to understand how you can feel bloated and hungry at the same time. But when you understand the importance of nutrients, it's easy to see that you can fill yourself to bursting on junk food and still be crying out for something nutritious.

The digestive process can be extremely energy sapping. It uses up more energy than any other activity, but we tend not to be aware of this because it goes on silently inside us while we're concentrating on other things. But have you ever noticed how much time carnivores spend asleep? They need the rest to digest all that meat. And for the same reason we all tend to fall asleep after Christmas dinner!

By contrast, fruit leaves us bounding with energy because

we use up so little digesting it. Junk food is hard to digest and dispose of and, therefore, uses up a lot of energy. When you try to satisfy your hunger by filling up with junk food, you deplete your energy reserves and fail to obtain the nutrients your body needs. A continuing hunger and growing lack of energy lead to one thing: a desire to eat more. But if all you eat is more of the same, the problem just gets worse. This is the vicious circle that leads us to put on weight.

YOU GAIN WEIGHT WHEN CONSUMPTION IS GREATER THAN DISPOSAL

It's as simple as that.

TENTH INSTRUCTION: TRY TO SATISFY YOUR HUNGER WITH REAL FOOD, NOT JUNK

This is the key to solving your weight problem with Easyway. Understand that overeating is brought about by eating the wrong foods and the door to your prison will swing open.

You'll notice I'm not telling you exactly what you can and can't eat. You have a Junk Margin so, like the chimp, there are no restrictions on what you eat. But if you try to satisfy your hunger with real food as often as you can, you'll quickly see the benefits, and as you go on you'll almost certainly find that the appeal of junk food diminishes and will eventually disappear altogether.

But you don't have to wait for that time to feel free. You can use the Junk Margin to make life easier for now, just as long as you understand that you won't satisfy your hunger unless you take in the vitamins, minerals, and energy that your body requires.

SUMMARY

- Fruit ticks all the boxes: looks good, smells good, feels good, tastes good.

- Fruit provides all our favorite flavors.

- Fruit is the easiest food for us to digest.

- Fruit gives us an energy surplus.

- Processing food kills nutrients, adds toxins, and diminishes water content.

- Tenth instruction: TRY TO SATISFY YOUR HUNGER WITH REAL FOOD, NOT JUNK.

Chapter 18

BEGIN THE DAY WELL

IN THIS CHAPTER
• *WHAT WE'VE ESTABLISHED* • *A CHANGE OF ROUTINE*
• *COMBINING FOODS* • *THE IDEAL BREAKFAST*
• *MAKE IT EASY ON YOURSELF*

It's time to take your first steps toward a new life of enjoyable, healthy eating, starting with the first meal of the day.

At the beginning of this book we made a claim, which you may have thought sounded too good to be true:

You can achieve your ideal weight easily, painlessly, and permanently, without having to diet or undergo special exercise, and without having to use willpower or feel deprived. In fact, you can eat as much of your favorite foods as you want, whenever you want.

Since reading that claim you've come a long way and, if you've followed all the instructions, you will have changed your perception of the way you eat and the way Nature intended you to eat.

• You know which foods really taste the best: fresh fruit, vegetables, nuts, and seeds, which are all good to eat without requiring any processing, including cooking. You also know that these are the foods that are ideally suited to the human digestive system, yielding all the nutrients we need and a net energy gain. There's no doubt that these are our favorite foods.

• You know which foods to avoid: processed foods, especially meat and dairy and those containing refined sugar. Meat and dairy are not suited to the human digestive system and the supposed nutritional benefits—protein, calcium, etc.—are far outweighed by the harm they cause and can be obtained much more efficiently from natural foods.

• You know when to eat: when you feel true hunger. You understand about the false hunger created by triggers such as a smell, or the addictive craving for refined sugar. All you have to do is follow Mother Nature's Guide and wait until your fuel gauge is indicating true hunger. Food tastes much better when you're truly hungry.

• You know when to stop eating: when your hunger is satisfied. You understand the importance of eating slowly, to give your body time to register the fact that it's received the nutrients it needs. You also understand that if you fill up on junk foods that don't provide the nutrients you need, you'll never satisfy your hunger.

• You know that there's no need to set yourself an ideal weight. Wild animals don't have an ideal weight in mind, yet they are never overweight. You can still use your scales to keep track of your progress and give yourself the encouragement of seeing your weight fall, but you'll know when you've achieved your ideal weight because you'll be able to look at yourself naked in the mirror and be happy with what you see.

• You know that dieting doesn't work and that relying on willpower to change your eating habits means consigning yourself to a lifetime of feeling deprived and miserable. By following Easyway, you won't feel deprived or miserable, because you'll be able to enjoy every meal and reap the benefits of good health and energy that come with eating the right foods.

Any doubts you may have had at the beginning of this book have now been replaced with knowledge. You've opened your mind and accepted that there is another side to the story, contrary to the brainwashing that you've been subjected to from birth. You can now see through the illusion and the myth that junk food gives you some sort of pleasure or crutch. Now to put all that knowledge into practice.

A NATURAL ROUTINE

The routine of eating three meals a day ties in roughly with our hunger patterns and, therefore, you could say that it's a healthy routine. But the purpose of this eating timetable has been lost. We eat in accordance with the clock, not with our hunger. Perhaps you think that breakfast time, lunch time and supper time are the times when you feel hungry, and that might well be the case if we weren't inclined to snack between meals, but our tendency to graze means that we're seldom truly hungry when it comes to lunch and supper time.

You need to reset your routine in accordance with your hunger. This won't be a problem; in fact, you'll find it very easy. Hunger is very flexible: you don't have to rush to satisfy it as soon as you feel those first slight pangs. You can live with it for hours without any discomfort at all, so if you find yourself feeling true hunger at a time when you can't eat—for example, during work—it's easy to wait until your next break and satisfy your hunger then. Remember, the longer you leave hunger to build up, the better your food will taste.

Some people think it's in their nature to pick at food all day like a grazing animal, but human beings were not designed to graze. Chimpanzees don't graze, sheep do. Which do you think is more closely related to humans? The reason people feel the need to graze is because they're permanently hungry—and that's because they're eating the wrong types of foods. They're not giving their body the nutrients it needs. Start eating the foods that were designed for you and you'll find that the desire to keep grazing soon disappears.

You also need to take control of the quantity of food you eat at each meal. That's the other problem with the routine of three meals a day: not only is the timing set by the clock, the quantity is set by conditioning. Neither of these is a response to what your body needs. Pay attention to your hunger and eat enough to satisfy it and no more.

From now on you're going to make the timing, volume, and content of your meals suit your own selfish needs.

MIXING AND MATCHING

We can learn a lot from the French when it comes to eating. They're world renowned for their culinary expertise, which stems from a genuine love of mealtimes. They don't sideline eating as a boring necessity to be dealt with while watching TV; they make an occasion of their meals, enjoy the social aspect of eating together, and pay much closer attention to the food on their plate. They also happen to have one of the lowest rates of heart disease in the world.

The French tend to take much longer over their meals and they like to separate different types of food into different courses. For example, they'll eat a salad course, then perhaps a meat course, then a vegetable course, and so on. This is a traditional way of eating that goes back way before our modern fascination with junk food and the concept of cramming an entire meal into a bun. The French way of eating is far more in touch with Mother Nature's Guide than the English and American way. It harks back to a time when we ate according to our needs, rather than a rigid routine.

Separating foods out as the French do takes the strain off your digestive system. While we're capable of digesting many different types of food—some much better than others—we're not able to cope efficiently with different foods at the same time. In order to digest protein, for example, the stomach will produce acidic juices, while the digestive juices for breaking down carbohydrates are alkaline. Mix an acid with an alkali and they neutralize each other.

So if the stomach is presented with meat (protein) and potatoes (carbohydrate) at the same time, its digestive juices will be neutralized and it will not be able to digest either.

The stomach will work overtime to keep producing acidic and alkaline juices and you'll feel the effects as indigestion and heartburn. After about eight hours it will admit defeat and pass the decomposing mass of badly combined foods on to the intestines. But it's too late for them to extract any nutritional value from it and they're merely saddled with the problem of passing this stodgy, toxic mass out of your system. That's no easy task. Food takes an average of 25 to 32 hours to pass through the digestive system and out of the body. When meat is involved that time can be doubled. That's a lot of time expending a lot of energy on something that is doing you no good whatsoever. And it can be very painful.

You might think you're being good by having just a piece of fruit for pudding after this mix-and-match main course, but if you add fruit to this bubbling concoction, it will also remain undigested and will just become part of the stagnant mass inside you. It will not be able to pass quickly into the intestines as it should do and its nutrients will not be absorbed.

You can easily avoid this unpalatable situation by following the French example and separating out the constituent parts of your meals, with time for a good chat in between.

- Eat fruit on its own or only with fresh salad and vegetables, not with meat or diary.
- Avoid mixing proteins with carbohydrates.
- Nonstarchy vegetables can be mixed with either proteins (meat and dairy) or carbohydrates (starchy vegetables such as potatoes, plus rice, pasta, and grains). This is because their high water content makes them digestible by both acidic and alkaline juices.

Follow these guidelines and you'll find every meal leaves you feeling energized and comfortable. You can still eat the occasional portion of fried fish in batter as part of your Junk Margin—just avoid those repulsive, fatty, stodgy fries that'll just make you feel bloated and awful. That's the beauty of this method—it doesn't require you to sacrifice anything. Just make sure these meals with Junk Margin items like that don't become the norm.

THE IDEAL BREAKFAST

To get the maximum benefit from fresh fruit, you need to digest it on its own. You should also allow at least half an hour before you eat any other type of food. You have the perfect opportunity to do this every day by eating fruit, and only fruit, for breakfast. The conditions are perfect: You won't have eaten since the previous evening; your stomach will be empty and ready to make the most of the fresh, juicy, delicious, thirst-quenching, nutrient- and energy-packed fruit; it will leave you completely satisfied and you won't feel the need to eat again for several hours.

Breakfast is most people's favorite meal of the day because it comes after our longest spell without food and in many people's minds there's nothing more enticing on weekends than a nice brunch. But after a few days of eating a fresh fruit breakfast, you begin to see the greasy combination of egg, bacon, waffles, etc. as exactly that: a mass of greasy, indigestible junk. That's how easy it is to reverse the brainwashing.

A fresh fruit breakfast also offers an unrivaled opportunity for variety. You might think you have a huge choice in the cereal aisle of your local supermarket, but aren't most of those options just the same thing molded into different shapes, sprinkled with sugar and all tasting pretty much the same? Head over to the fruit section and look at your options. You'll find at least 20 different fresh fruits, all with their own distinct flavor, all in their natural state, ready to eat, smelling delicious, and looking fantastic.

YOU CAN EAT AS MANY FRUITS AS YOU WANT AND YOU WON'T PUT ON WEIGHT

15,504

If you have 20 different fruits to choose from and you want to eat a combination of five for breakfast, this is the number of different combinations available to you. That's a different breakfast every day for over 42 years!

As long as you make a fresh fruit breakfast the norm, you can still eat the occasional cooked breakfast or bowl of cereal (if you feel like it) without upsetting your new healthy, energetic routine. The Junk Margin allows for it. With Easyway there are no restrictions, no feelings of deprivation and misery—only health, energy, and joy!

KEEP IT SIMPLE

ELEVENTH INSTRUCTION: EAT FRUIT AND ONLY FRUIT FOR BREAKFAST

You'll find it easy to change to a fresh fruit breakfast if you don't try to change all of your other eating habits at the same time. Starting with breakfast is an ideal way to ease yourself into your new routine and it's made all the easier by the absence of any restrictions on what you eat during the rest of the day.

You might find this approach surprisingly lax. We get the same reaction from smokers when we tell them to keep smoking as usual until given the instruction to smoke their final cigarette. This method is called Easyway for a reason. If you have to change your whole way of eating at a stroke, you'll put unnecessary pressure on yourself and it will become anything but easy. Now that you've begun to change your mindset and unravel the brainwashing, there's no rush to reach a certain goal: your goal was achieved the moment you took your first step. You don't have to wait for anything to happen. You can start enjoying a much healthier and more pleasurable way of eating immediately.

Just take one step at a time and gradually change the types of food you eat to those that are best for you. It's an easy change to make because those are the foods that taste the best and once you get into the routine of eating them, you'll find that they become your favorites. Unlike a diet, which you leap into wholeheartedly but then give up on as your willpower runs out, Easyway is a method that you can take at your own pace, knowing that you've already solved your problem simply by starting to change.

So take your time to feel completely at ease with that first step of eating fruit and only fruit for breakfast before you move on to other meals. If you don't, there's a danger that you'll start craving certain dishes and relying on willpower to combat the craving. It will soon feel like a diet and ultimately it will fail.

After eating fruit and only fruit for breakfast for a few days, it will become second nature—or rather first nature. This is the ideal food designed for all of us and as you rediscover the pleasure of eating that delicious variety of juicy, nutrient-packed, high-water-content fruits and think about the ease with which you're going to digest it and the benefits you're going to derive from it, you'll soon wonder why you ever ate anything else for breakfast.

Very soon you'll begin to feel those benefits. Your weight will come down and you'll feel more energetic. You'll also find breakfast a genuine pleasure.

As you realize that the method is working and it really is easy, you'll feel confident that it will go on working and being easy.

Just changing what you eat for breakfast is enough to make

that difference. While this is happening you can start applying the counter-brainwashing techniques I've described to meat, dairy, and chocolate and see what healthy, natural foods you can find to replace them. Buoyed up by the success of your new breakfast routine, you will be champing at the bit to try all sorts of nutritious foods and see how they benefit you.

But remember to keep it steady and make it easy. You have the rest of your life ahead of you and there'll be plenty of signs that you've got your weight problem cracked. Your scales will show you that the pounds are falling off. Your mirror will show you that the unsightly lumps are disappearing. Your stomach will tell you that it's finding life a lot easier now that you're giving it a nice, easy start to the day. And your energy levels will tell you that you're getting more benefit from your food than ever before.

This is more than most women hope for when they first pick up this book. The primary objective is to lose weight, but you understand now that losing weight and achieving your ideal weight is a consequence of eating correctly as a response to your natural instincts, not as a diet. A further change that people don't bargain for is that you develop a preference for natural healthy foods and a growing number of processed foods now turn you off.

This is the preference given to us by nature. It's a clear indication that you're unraveling the brainwashing and your progress is unstoppable.

SUMMARY

• Let hunger dictate the timing, quantity, and content of your meals.

• Learn the combinations that make digestion easier.

• Try to avoid the combination of protein and carbohydrate as much as possible.

• Eleventh instruction: EAT FRUIT AND ONLY FRUIT FOR BREAKFAST.

• Take it one step at a time—nothing can stop you now!

Chapter 19

ENJOY THE LIFE YOU DESERVE

> ## IN THIS CHAPTER
> - *A RECIPE FOR HAPPINESS*
> - *EXERCISE FOR PLEASURE*
> - *THE MOMENT OF TRUTH*

Congratulations! You've escaped the junk trap forever. Now you can get on with enjoying life right away, just as nature intended.

In Chapter One, I looked at the reasons women want to lose weight and concluded that the most powerful reason was to free yourself from the misery of having no control over your eating. Being overweight has a negative impact on the way you look and the way you feel, and of course the two are closely connected. It also has a potentially serious impact on your health, which can cause its own worries. But the worst aspect of all is facing each meal, every day of your life, with a sense of dread, helplessness, or even self-loathing, knowing that the food you eat is going to make your condition worse.

We were not designed by nature to dread eating. On the contrary, we were designed to enjoy it. Everything we do for our own genuine benefit leaves us feeling happy—that's Mother Nature's design to insure we continue to seek out the things we need to survive and thrive.

Although you picked up this book in the hope of finding a method to help you lose weight, the real aim of the book is to help you find the happiness you're designed to get from life. By nature you will eat two or three meals every day for the rest of your life. That's a lot of opportunities for happiness. All you have to do is eat the foods that were designed by Nature to make you happy. And as a consequence of eating correctly, you'll also achieve your ideal weight.

The reason most weight-loss methods ultimately fail is because they take the pleasure out of mealtimes. The beauty of this method is it puts the pleasure back into mealtimes and helps you lose weight as a consequence. It's a win–win. When you first read the claim at the start of the book, you may have thought it sounded too good to be true. We're bombarded with misinformation that losing weight has to be hard. How can any weight-loss method be a win–win? But that's the way Mother Nature designed it to be.

We're not designed by nature to be overweight and miserable, nor to sacrifice genuine pleasures, or put ourselves through programs of self-punishment. Genuine pleasure comes from the things in life that make us stronger individually and collectively: eating nutritious food, exercising for pleasure, socializing, dancing, singing, reproducing… In short, Nature created us to enjoy ourselves and be happy. It's only by trying to outsmart Nature that we've lost sight of this truth.

EXERCISE FOR PLEASURE

Exercise is not the way to lose weight, but your body, like that of every animal on Earth, was designed to be exercised. We're lucky that our intelligence has spared us the need to burn energy looking for food and come up with far more enjoyable ways to exercise.

The cycle of healthy eating and exercise is not something you have to work at. You'll feel it working for you right from the start. Your weight will go down as you're no longer overloading your body with unwanted junk. You will feel healthier and your energy levels will rise. You won't have to force yourself to take exercise; you'll be champing at the bit to get out there. Just make sure that the exercise is enjoyable. You're spoilt for choice. Avoid all those miserable machines that are designed to imprison you in your house or the gym, going nowhere, and get outdoors. It can be anything from bowling to bungee jumping.

And when you feel hungry afterward, you'll know that it means you'll have a good appetite for your next meal, the food will taste delicious, and you'll relish every mouthful without any sense of guilt whatsoever. You'll also feel yourself getting stronger. Your muscles and lungs will benefit and your capacity for exercise will increase. Before long you'll find yourself looking in the mirror and being very happy with what you see.

Your choice of recreation will also have social benefits, giving your life purpose and pleasure, and removing the boredom, which is a major trigger for eating junk.

THE MOMENT OF TRUTH

Easyway isn't a diet. It's a method designed for life and it sets you free from the moment you reverse the brainwashing and start seeing the truth about your favorite foods and the foods that belong in the Junk Margin. You don't have to wait until you've reached some target weight before you can say you've succeeded. You've already succeeded by following all the instructions.

But it can be helpful to draw a line in the sand so that you can say, "This is the moment I walked free." With smokers I have the ritual of the final cigarette. Having encouraged them to keep smoking throughout the book, I then ask them to smoke one last time, concentrating on the taste, the smell, the brown residue on the filter that transfers itself to their lips and lungs, and to make a solemn vow never to smoke again. In most cases, they've already changed their mindset and have no desire to smoke whatsoever, but this ritual confirms everything they now know and gives them a reference point for the future, should they ever need reminding of the elation they felt when they realized they were free from the trap.

Hopefully you're feeling a similar sense of excitement at the life that awaits you, free from the slavery to junk food. Although you're already free and can start enjoying life immediately, this would be a good time to go through your own ritual. Unlike smoking, you're not vowing to quit junk food altogether, but you are fixing in your mind the knowledge that the foods you used to regard as your favorites are actually not the foods designed to give you most pleasure.

You can reinforce this fact in your mind by going through a similar ritual to the final cigarette. Whatever your favorite food used to be, make yourself eat it, preferably between meals when you're not truly hungry. Take the time to smell it and focus on how it feels in your hand. Does it look good? Take a bite and feel it in your mouth as you chew. What are you tasting? Is there a genuine flavour there, or is it the sweetness of refined sugar that's the overriding sensation? If there is a flavor, is it the flavor of fruit? Strip away the taste and what are you left with? Is that something you want to swallow down into your stomach?

You don't have to finish the food. Often one mouthful is enough. When you've had enough, remind yourself of everything you've learned about junk food and fix in your mind that this is not your favorite food. Congratulate yourself on getting free from the junk food trap. You've opened your mind and seen the truth behind the illusions sold to us by the food industry. You've given yourself back the power to make your own decisions about the food you eat.

YOU'RE IN CONTROL

CONCLUSION

Eating junk food creates a painful clash between guilt and self-deprivation. You feel guilty for eating too much and deprived because you know you can't eat as much as you want to.

Eating natural, healthy food creates a harmonious balance between intake, exercise, and appetite. Each element provides for the next and each is a pleasure with wonderful added benefits. The net result is self-perpetuating health and happiness. And it tastes so much better.

In the first case, life always seems hard. In the latter, life is easy. There's nothing unnatural or forced about it. Ninety-nine percent of animals enjoy eating their favorite foods every day without even having to think about it. Nature has provided them with the instinctive tools to survive and thrive. Why should we be any different?

Congratulations on being free. Enjoy your life free from the nightmare of eating junk. Remember—you haven't given up anything—you've got rid of a disease. Celebrate now—you're already free.

Chapter 20

USEFUL REMINDERS

Here's a summary of the key points that we've discussed, together with a reminder of the instructions. You might find it useful to refer back to these points from time to time.

THE INSTRUCTIONS

• Animals eat when they're hungry and stop eating when their hunger is satisfied—not when they're full. Humans in the developed world have been conditioned to eat because it's a certain time of day, or they're bored, or they've been brainwashed to believe that the food before them will give them pleasure, regardless of whether they're hungry. This conditioning and brainwashing is easy to reverse.

• The real purpose of eating is to fuel your body with the energy and nutrients it requires to remain healthy and strong.

• Hunger is the signal that your body is running low and needs refueling. Hunger gives you the appetite that makes food taste better. Therefore, hunger is the key to enjoyable eating. Stay in touch with your hunger, avoid eating when you're not hungry, and make hunger the basis of your eating routine.

- You can't satisfy hunger with junk food. Hunger is only satisfied when the body gets the nutrients it needs. If you try to fill up on junk food, you'll remain hungry even when you're full. This is the cause of overeating.

- Beware of the convention for loading people's plates with more food than they need. If you really care about the people you're cooking for, give them a well-proportioned plate of good, healthy, nutritious food. And if someone serves you more food than you have an appetite for, just don't eat it. Monitor your hunger and stop eating when you've had enough. It's not impolite.

- Beware the custom for putting out nibbles before a meal. There's nothing sociable about laying a trap for your guests that will lure them into overeating. The salt and sugar in these snacks causes an addictive craving that leads to excessive consumption and any nutritional value is negligible.

- Watch out for all processed foods. If a food has to be tampered with in any way to make it edible, then it's not designed for human consumption.

- Beware the con of refined sugar, which fools our taste buds into thinking we're eating the sweet-tasting food that was designed for us when, in fact, we're eating poison.

- Base your eating habits on the knowledge that the foods that taste best are the high-water-content foods that are best for you, and free your taste buds from the brainwashing of the junk food industry.

THE INSTRUCTIONS

1   FOLLOW ALL THE INSTRUCTIONS IN ORDER

2   KEEP AN OPEN MIND

3   START OFF WITH A FEELING OF ELATION

4   DISPENSE WITH ANY TARGET WEIGHT

5   IGNORE ANY ADVICE THAT CONFLICTS WITH MOTHER NATURE'S GUIDE

6   NEVER DOUBT YOUR DECISION TO QUIT

7   IGNORE ANY ADVICE THAT CONFLICTS WITH EASYWAY

8   GO FOR IT!

9   AVOID EATING UNLESS YOU'RE HUNGRY

10 TRY TO SATISFY YOUR HUNGER WITH REAL FOOD,
    NOT JUNK

11 EAT FRUIT AND ONLY FRUIT FOR BREAKFAST

LIST OF ALLEN CARR'S EASYWAY CENTERS

The following list indicates the countries where Allen Carr's Easyway To Stop Smoking Centers are currently operational.

Check www.allencarr.com for latest additions to this list.

The success rate at the centers, based on the three-month money-back guarantee, is over 90 per cent.

Selected centers also offer sessions that deal with alcohol, other drugs and weight issues. Please check with your nearest center, listed below, for details.

Allen Carr's Easyway guarantee that you will find it easy to stop at the centers or your money back.

JOIN US!

Allen Carr's Easyway Centers have spread throughout the world with incredible speed and success. Our global franchise network now covers more than 150 cities in over 45 countries. This amazing growth has been achieved entirely organically. Former addicts, just like you, were so impressed by the ease with which they stopped that they felt inspired to contact us to see how they could bring the method to their region.

If you feel the same, contact us for details on how to become an Allen Carr's Easyway To Stop Smoking or an Allen Carr's Easyway To Stop Drinking franchisee.

Email us at: **join-us@allencarr.com** including your full name, postal address and region of interest.

SUPPORT US!

No, don't send us money!

You have achieved something really marvellous. Every time we hear of someone escaping from the sinking ship, we get a feeling of enormous satisfaction.

It would give us great pleasure to hear that you have freed yourself from the slavery of addiction so please visit the following web page where you can tell us of your success, inspire others to follow in your footsteps and hear about ways you can help to spread the word.

www.allencarr.com/fanzone

You can "like" our facebook page here
www.facebook.com/AllenCarr

Together, we can help further Allen Carr's mission: to cure the world of addiction.

LONDON CENTER AND WORLDWIDE HEAD OFFICE

Park House, 14 Pepys Road,
Raynes Park, London SW20 8NH
Tel: +44 (0)20 8944 7761
Fax: +44 (0)20 8944 8619
Email: mail@allencarr.com
Website: www.allencarr.com
Therapists: John Dicey, Colleen
Dwyer, Crispin Hay, Emma Hudson,
Rob Fielding, Sam Kelser, Rob Groves,
Debbie Brewer-West, Duncan Bhaskaran-
Brown, Gerry Williams (alcohol), Monique
Douglas (Weight)

Worldwide Press Office

Contact: John Dicey
Tel: +44 (0)7970 88 44 52
Email: media@allencarr.com

CANADA

Sessions held throughout Canada
Email: mail@allencarr.com
Website: www.allencarr.com

USA

Sessions held throughout the USA
Toll free: 855 440 3777
Email: support@usa.allencarr.com
Website: www.allencarr.com

New York

Toll free: 855 440 3777
Therapists: Natalie Clays and Team
Email: support@usa.allencarr.com
Website: www.allencarr.com

Los Angeles

Toll free: 855 440 3777
Therapists: Natalie Clays and Team
Email: support@usa.allencarr.com
Website: www.allencarr.com

Milwaukee (and South Wisconsin)

Tel: +1 262 770 1260
Therapist: Wayne Spaulding
Email: wayne@easywaywisconsin.com
Website: www.allencarr.com

UK CENTERS

Birmingham

Tel & Fax: 0800 389 2115
Therapists: John Dicey, Colleen
Dwyer, Crispin Hay, Emma Hudson,
Rob Fielding, Sam Kelser, Rob Groves,
Debbie Brewer-West, Gerry Williams
(alcohol)
Email: mail@allencarr.com
Website: www.allencarr.com

Bournemouth

Tel: 0800 389 2115
Therapists: John Dicey, Colleen Dwyer,
Crispin Hay, Emma Hudson,
Rob Fielding, Sam Kelser, Rob Groves,
Debbie Brewer-West
Email: mail@allencarr.com
Website: www.allencarr.com

Brentwood

Tel: 0800 389 2115
Therapists: John Dicey, Colleen Dwyer,
Crispin Hay, Emma Hudson,
Rob Fielding, Sam Kelser, Rob Groves,
Debbie Brewer-West
Email: mail@allencarr.com
Website: www.allencarr.com

Brighton

Tel: 0800 389 2115
Therapists: John Dicey, Colleen Dwyer,
Crispin Hay, Emma Hudson,
Rob Fielding, Sam Kelser, Rob Groves,
Debbie Brewer-West
Email: mail@allencarr.com
Website: www.allencarr.com

Bristol

Tel: 0800 389 2115
Therapists: John Dicey, Colleen Dwyer,
Crispin Hay, Emma Hudson,
Rob Fielding, Sam Kelser, Rob Groves,
Debbie Brewer-West
Email: mail@allencarr.com
Website: www.allencarr.com

Cambridge
Tel: 0800 389 2115
Therapists: John Dicey, Colleen Dwyer,
Crispin Hay, Emma Hudson, Rob Fielding,
Sam Kelser, Rob Groves, Debbie Brewer-West
Email: mail@allencarr.com
Website: www.allencarr.com

Coventry
Tel: 0800 321 3007
Therapist: Rob Fielding
Email: info@easywaymidlands.co.uk
Website: www.allencarr.com

Cumbria
Tel: 0800 077 6187
Therapist: Mark Keen
Email: mark@easywaymanchester.co.uk
Website: www.allencarr.com

Derby
Tel: 0800 389 2115
Therapist: John Dicey, Colleen Dwyer,
Crispin Hay, Emma Hudson,
Rob Fielding, Sam Kelser, Rob Groves,
Debbie Brewer-West
Email: mail@allencarr.com
Website: www.allencarr.com

Guernsey
Tel: 0800 077 6187
Therapist: Mark Keen
Email: mark@easywaymanchester.co.uk
Website: www.allencarr.com

Isle of Man
Tel: 0800 077 6187
Therapist: Mark Keen
Email: mark@easywaymanchester.co.uk
Website: www.allencarr.com

Jersey
Tel: 0800 077 6187
Therapist: Mark Keen
Email: mark@easywaymanchester.co.uk
Website: www.allencarr.com

Kent
Tel: 0800 389 2115
Therapists: John Dicey, Colleen Dwyer,
Crispin Hay, Emma Hudson,
Rob Fielding, Sam Kelser, Rob Groves,
Debbie Brewer-West
Email: mail@allencarr.com
Website: www.allencarr.com

Lancashire
Tel: 0800 077 6187
Therapist: Mark Keen
Email: mark@easywaymanchester.co.uk
Website: www.allencarr.com

Leeds
Tel: 0800 077 6187
Therapist: Mark Keen
Email: mark@easywaymanchester.co.uk
Website: www.allencarr.com

Leicester
Tel: 0800 321 3007
Therapist: Rob Fielding
Email: info@easywaymidlands.co.uk
Website: www.allencarr.com

Lincoln
Tel: 0800 321 3007
Therapist: Rob Fielding
Email: info@easywaymidlands.co.uk
Website: www.allencarr.com

Liverpool
Tel: 0800 077 6187
Therapist: Mark Keen
Email: mark@easywaymanchester.co.uk
Website: www.allencarr.com

Manchester
Tel: 0800 077 6187
Therapist: Mark Keen
Email: mark@easywaymanchester.co.uk
Website: www.allencarr.com

Manchester—alcohol sessions
Tel: +44 (0)7936 712942
Therapist: Mike Connolly
Email: info@stopdrinkingnorth.co.uk
Website: www.allencarr.com

Milton Keynes
Tel: 0800 389 2115
Therapists: John Dicey, Colleen Dwyer,
Crispin Hay, Emma Hudson,
Rob Fielding, Sam Kelser, Rob Groves,
Debbie Brewer-West
Email: mail@allencarr.com
Website: www.allencarr.com

Newcastle/North East
Tel: 0800 077 6187
Therapist: Mark Keen
Email: mark@easywaymanchester.co.uk
Website: www.allencarr.com

Northern Ireland/Belfast
Tel: 0800 077 6187
Therapist: Mark Keen
Email: mark@easywaymanchester.co.uk
Website: www.allencarr.com

Nottingham
Tel: 0800 389 2115
Therapist: John Dicey, Colleen Dwyer,
Crispin Hay, Emma Hudson, Rob Fielding,
Sam Kelser, Rob Groves, Debbie Brewer-
West
Email: mail@allencarr.com
Website: www.allencarr.com

Oxford
Tel: 0800 389 2115
Therapists: John Dicey, Colleen Dwyer,
Crispin Hay, Emma Hudson, Rob Fielding,
Sam Kelser, Rob Groves, Debbie Brewer-West
Email: mail@allencarr.com
Website: www.allencarr.com

Reading
Tel: 0800 389 2115
Therapists: John Dicey, Colleen Dwyer,
Crispin Hay, Emma Hudson, Rob Fielding,
Sam Kelser, Rob Groves, Debbie Brewer-West
Email: mail@allencarr.com
Website: www.allencarr.com

SCOTLAND
Glasgow and Edinburgh
Tel: +44 (0)131 449 7858
Therapists: Paul Melvin and Jim McCreadie
Email: info@easywayscotland.co.uk
Website: www.allencarr.com

Southampton
Tel: 0800 389 2115
Therapists: John Dicey, Colleen Dwyer,
Crispin Hay, Emma Hudson,
Rob Fielding, Sam Kelser, Rob Groves,
Debbie Brewer-West
Email: mail@allencarr.com
Website: www.allencarr.com

Southport
Tel: 0800 077 6187
Therapist: Mark Keen
Email: mark@easywaymanchester.co.uk
Website: www.allencarr.com

Staines/Heathrow
Tel: 0800 389 2115
Therapists: John Dicey, Colleen Dwyer,
Crispin Hay, Emma Hudson, Rob Fielding,
Sam Kelser, Rob Groves, Debbie Brewer-West
Email: mail@allencarr.com
Website: www.allencarr.com

Stevenage
Tel: 0800 389 2115
Therapists: John Dicey, Colleen Dwyer,
Crispin Hay, Emma Hudson, Rob Fielding,
Sam Kelser, Rob Groves, Debbie Brewer-West
Email: mail@allencarr.com
Website: www.allencarr.com

Stoke
Tel: 0800 389 2115
Therapist: John Dicey, Colleen Dwyer,
Crispin Hay, Emma Hudson, Rob Fielding,
Sam Kelser, Rob Groves, Debbie Brewer-West
Email: mail@allencarr.com
Website: www.allencarr.com

Surrey
Park House, 14 Pepys Road, Raynes Park,
London SW20 8NH
Tel: +44 (0)20 8944 7761
Fax: +44 (0)20 8944 8619
Therapists: John Dicey, Colleen
Dwyer, Crispin Hay, Emma Hudson,
Rob Fielding, Sam Kelser, Rob Groves,
Debbie Brewer-West, Duncan Bhaskaran-
Brown, Gerry Williams (alcohol), Monique
Douglas (Weight)
Email: mail@allencarr.com
Website: www.allencarr.com

Watford
Tel: 0800 389 2115
Therapists: John Dicey, Colleen Dwyer,
Crispin Hay, Emma Hudson, Rob Fielding,
Sam Kelser, Rob Groves, Debbie Brewer-West
Email: mail@allencarr.com
Website: www.allencarr.com

Worcester
Tel: 0800 321 3007
Therapist: Rob Fielding
Email: info@easywaymidlands.co.uk
Website: www.allencarr.com

WORLDWIDE CENTERS

AUSTRALIA
ACT, NSW, NT, QLD, VIC
Tel: 1300 848 028
Therapist: Natalie Clays and Team
Email: natalie@allencarr.com.au
Website: www.allencarr.com

South Australia
Tel: 1300 848 028
Therapist: Jaime Reed
Email: sa@allencarr.com.au
Website: www.allencarr.com

Western Australia
Tel: 1300 848 028
Therapist: Natalie Clays and Team
Email: natalie@allencarr.com.au
Website: www.allencarr.com

AUSTRIA
Sessions held throughout Austria
Freephone: 0800RAUCHEN
(0800 7282436)
Tel: +43 (0)3512 44755
Therapists: Erich Kellermann and Team
Email: info@allen-carr.at
Website: www.allencarr.com

BAHRAIN
Please check website for details
Website: www.allencarr.com

BELGIUM
Antwerp
Tel: +32 (0)3 281 6255
Fax: +32 (0)3 744 0608
Therapist: Dirk Nielandt
Email: info@allencarr.be
Website: www.allencarr.com

BRAZIL
Therapist : Lilian Brunstein
Email: lilian@easywaysp.com.br
Website: www.allencarr.com

BULGARIA
Tel: 0800 14104 / +359 899 88 99 07
Therapist: Rumyana Kostadinova
Email: rk@nepushaveche.com
Website: www.allencarr.com

CHILE
Tel: +56 2 4744587
Therapist: Claudia Sarmiento
Email: contacto@allencarr.cl
Website: www.allencarr.com

CYPRUS
Please check website for details
Email: mail@allencarr.com
Website: www.allencarr.com

DENMARK
Sessions held throughout Denmark
Tel: +45 70267711
Therapist: Mette Fønss
Email: mette@easyway.dk
Website: www.allencarr.com

ESTONIA
Tel: +372 733 0044
Therapist: Henry Jakobson
Email: info@allencarr.ee
Website: www.allencarr.com

FINLAND
Tel: +358-(0)45 3544099
Therapist: Janne Ström
Email: info@allencarr.fi
Website: www.allencarr.com

FRANCE
Sessions held throughout France
Freephone: 0800 386387
Tel: +33 (4)91 33 54 55
Therapists: Erick Serre and Team
Email: info@allencarr.fr
Website: www.allencarr.com

GERMANY
Sessions held throughout Germany
Freephone: 08000RAUCHEN
(0800 07282436)
Tel: +49 (0) 8031 90190-0
Therapists: Erich Kellermann and Team
Email: info@allen-carr.de
Website: www.allencarr.com

GREECE
Sessions held throughout Greece
Tel: +30 210 5224087
Therapist: Panos Tzouras
Email: panos@allencarr.gr
Website: www.allencarr.com

GUATEMALA
Tel: +502 2362 0000
Therapist: Michelle Binford
Email: bienvenid@dejedefumarfacil.com
Website: www.allencarr.com

HONG KONG
Email: info@easywayhongkong.com
Website: www.allencarr.com

HUNGARY
Seminars in Budapest and
12 other cities across Hungary
Tel: 06 80 624 426 (freephone) or
+36 20 580 9244
Therapist: Gábor Szász
Email: szasz.gabor@allencarr.hu
Website: www.allencarr.com

INDIA
Bangalore and Chennai
Tel: +91 (0)80 4154 0624
Therapist: Suresh Shottam
Email: info@easywaytostopsmoking.co.in
Website: www.allencarr.com

IRAN
Please check website for details
Website: www.allencarr.com

ISRAEL
Sessions held throughout Israel
Tel: +972 (0)3 6212525
Therapists: Ramy Romanovsky,
Orit Rozen
Email: info@allencarr.co.il
Website: www.allencarr.com

ITALY
Sessions held throughout Italy
Tel/Fax: +39 (0)2 7060 2438
Therapists: Francesca Cesati
and Team
Email: info@easywayitalia.com
Website: www.allencarr.com

JAPAN
Sessions held throughout Japan
www.allencarr.com

LEBANON
Tel: +961 1 791 5565
Therapist: Sadek El-Assaad
Email: info@AllenCarrEasyWay.me
Website: www.allencarr.com

MAURITIUS
Tel: +230 5727 5103
Therapist: Heidi Hoareau
Email: info@allencarr.mu
Website: www.allencarr.com

MEXICO
Sessions held throughout Mexico
Tel: +52 55 2623 0631
Therapists: Jorge Davo and Team
Email: info@allencarr-mexico.com
Website: www.allencarr.com

NETHERLANDS
Sessions held throughout the Netherlands
Allen Carr's Easyway
'stoppen met roken'
Tel: (+31)53 478 43 62 /
(+31)900 786 77 37
Email: info@allencarr.nl
Website: www.allencarr.com

NEW ZEALAND
North Island – Auckland
Tel: +64 (0)27 4139 381
Therapist: Natalie Clays and Team
Email: natalie@allencarr.co.nz
Website: www.allencarr.com

South Island – Wellington and Christchurch
Tel: +64 (0) 0800 848 028
Therapist: Natalie Clays and Team
Email: natalie@allencarr.co.nz

South Island – Dunedin and Invercargill
Tel: +64 (0)27 4139 381
Therapist: Debbie Kinder
Email: easywaysouth@icloud.com
Website: www.allencarr.com

NORWAY
Therapist: Laila Thorsen
Please check website for details
Website: www.allencarr.com

PERU
Lima
Tel: +511 637 7310
Therapist: Luis Loranca

Email: lloranca@dejardefumaraltoque.com
Website: www.allencarr.com

POLAND
Sessions held throughout Poland
Therapist: Michael Kochon
Tel : +48 (0) 22 621 36 11
Email: info@allen-carr.pl
Website: www.allencarr.com

POLAND – Alcohol sessions
Please check website for details
Website: www.allencarr.com

PORTUGAL
Oporto
Tel: +351 22 9958698
Therapist: Ria Slof
Email: info@comodeixardefumar.com
Website: www.allencarr.com

REPUBLIC OF IRELAND
Dublin
Tel: +353 (0)1 499 9010
Therapists: Paul Melvin & Jim McCreadie
Email: info@allencarr.ie
Website: www.allencarr.com

ROMANIA
Tel: +40 (0)7321 3 8383
Therapist: Cristina Nichita
Email: raspunsuri@allencarr.ro
Website: www.allencarr.com

RUSSIA
Allen Carr's Easyway to Stop Smoking
Live Seminars & Online Video Programme
Tel: +7 495 644 64 26
Freecall +7 (800) 250 6622
Therapist: Alexander Fomin
Email: info@allencarr.ru
Website: www.allencarr.com

Allen Carr's Easyway to Stop Drinking
Live Seminars & Online Video Programme
Tel: +8 (800) 302 80 68
+7 985 207 47 93
Therapist: Artem Kasyanov
Email: info@allencarrlife.ru
Website: www.allencarr.com

St Petersburg
Please check website for details
Website: www.allencarr.com

SAUDI ARABIA
Please check website for details
Website: www.allencarr.com

SERBIA
Belgrade
Tel: +381 (0)11 308 8686
Email: office@allencarr.co.rs
Website: www.allencarr.com

SINGAPORE
Tel: +65 62241450
Therapist: Pam Oei
Email: pam@allencarr.com.sg
Website: www.allencarr.com

SLOVENIA
Tel: 00386 (0)40 77 61 77
Therapist: Grega Server
Email: easyway@easyway.si
Website: www.allencarr.com

SOUTH AFRICA
Sessions held throughout South Africa
National Booking Line: 0861 100 200
Head Office: 15 Draper Square, Draper St,
Claremont 7708, Cape Town, Cape Town:
Dr Charles Nel
Tel: +27 (0)21 851 5883
Mobile: 083 600 5555
Therapists: Dr Charles Nel,
Malcolm Robinson and Team
Email: easyway@allencarr.co.za
Website: www.allencarr.com

SOUTH KOREA
Seoul
Tel: +82 (0)70 4227 1862
Therapist: Yousung Cha
Email: master@allencarr.co.kr
Website: www.allencarr.com

SPAIN
Tel: +34 910 05 29 99
Therapist: Luis Loranca
Email: informes@AllenCarrOfficial.es
Website: www.allencarr.com

SWEDEN
Tel: +46 70 695 6850
Therapists: Nina Ljungqvist,
Renée Johansson
Email: info@easyway.se
Website: www.allencarr.com

SWITZERLAND
Sessions held throughout Switzerland
Freephone: 0800RAUCHEN
(0800/728 2436)
Tel: +41 (0)52 383 3773
Fax: +41 (0)52 3833774
Therapists: Cyrill Argast and Team
For sessions in Suisse Romand
and Svizzera Italiana:
Tel: 0800 386 387
Email: info@allen-carr.ch
Website: www.allencarr.com

TURKEY
Sessions held throughout Turkey
Tel: +90 212 358 5307
Therapist: Emre Üstünuçar
Email: info@allencarrturkiye.com
Website: www.allencarr.com

UNITED ARAB EMIRATES
Dubai and Abu Dhabi
Tel: +971 56 693 4000
Therapist: Sadek El-Assaad
Email: info@AllenCarrEasyWay.me
Website: www.allencarr.com

OTHER ALLEN CARR PUBLICATIONS

Allen Carr's revolutionary Easyway method is available in a wide
variety of formats, including digitally as audiobooks and ebooks,
and has been successfully applied to a broad range of subjects.
For more information about Easyway publications, please visit
shop.allencarr.com

Good Sugar Bad Sugar

The Easy Way to Quit Sugar

The Easy Way to Lose Weight

No More Diets

Allen Carr's Easy Way to Quit
Smoking

The Easy Way to Quit Vaping

Allen Carr's Quit Smoking Boot
Camp

Your Personal Stop Smoking Plan

The Illustrated Easy Way to Stop
Smoking

Allen Carr's Easy Way for Women
to Quit Smoking

The Illustrated Easy Way for
Women to Stop Smoking

Finally Free!

Smoking Sucks (Parent Guide with
16 page pull-out comic)

The Little Book of Quitting Smoking

How to Be a Happy Nonsmoker

No More Ashtrays

The Only Way to Stop Smoking
Permanently

Allen Carr's Quit Drinking Without
Willpower

The Easy Way to Control Alcohol

Your Personal Stop Drinking Plan

The Illustrated Easy Way to Stop
Drinking

Allen Carr's Easy Way for Women
to Quit Drinking

No More Hangovers

Smart Phone Dumb Phone

The Easy Way to Mindfulness

The Easy Way to Stop Gambling

No More Gambling

No More Worrying

Get Out of Debt Now

No More Debt

No More Fear of Flying

The Easy Way to Quit Caffeine

Packing It In The Easy Way
(the autobiography)

Want Easyway on your **smartphone** or **tablet**?
Search for "Allen Carr" in your app store.

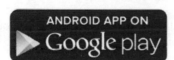 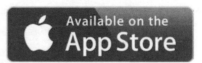

Easyway publications are also available as **audiobooks**.
Visit **shop.allencarr.com** to find out more.

 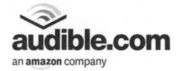

DISCOUNT VOUCHER
for
ALLEN CARR'S
EASYWAY CENTERS

Recover the price of this book when you attend an
Allen Carr's Easyway Center
anywhere in the world!

Allen Carr's Easyway has a global network of stop
smoking centers where we guarantee you'll find it easy
to stop smoking or your money back.

**The success rate based on this
unique money-back guarantee is over 90%.**

Sessions addressing weight, alcohol and other
drug addictions are also available at certain centers.

When you book your session, mention this
voucher and you'll receive a discount of
the price of this book. Contact your nearest
center for more information on how the sessions
work and to book your appointment.

**Details of Allen Carr's Easyway
Centers can be found at**

www.allencarr.com

This offer is not valid in conjunction with any other offer/promotion.